Practical Manual of Pleural Pathology

Angelo G. Casalini
Editor

Practical Manual of Pleural Pathology

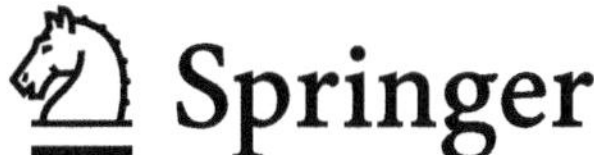
Springer

Editor
Angelo G. Casalini
Parma, Italy

ISBN 978-3-031-20314-5 ISBN 978-3-031-20312-1 (eBook)
https://doi.org/10.1007/978-3-031-20312-1

This Springer imprint is published by the registered company Springer Nature Switzerland AG
The registered company address is: Gewerbestrasse 11, 6330 Cham, Switzerland

This book is dedicated to all medical doctors who died and healthcare professionals who lost their lives during the SARS-CoV-2 pandemic.

Preface

This manual is the fruit of over 40 years of Pulmonology and Thoracic Endoscopy, about 900 medical thoracoscopies performed, the organisation of 33 theoretical-practical courses on Interventional Pulmonology at the Hospital of Parma, the participation of the authors as speakers and teachers at countless courses and conferences in Italy and abroad and the great collaboration with other Italian Pneumologists that have always dealt with Pleural Pathology.

The experience gained in this field, and in particular in Medical Thoracoscopy, is also derived from the repeated attendance of the authors at one of the most important international centres in this field: the Department of Pulmonology, Hôpital de la Conception, Marseilles, France, directed first by Prof. C. Boutin and later by Prof. Philippe Astoul.

The training and growth path followed by the Pulmonology—Thoracic Endoscopy Division of Parma Hospital has been shared with other Italian centres that have always dealt with this pathology and, over the years, this shared path has led to an increasingly in-depth mastery of the subject deriving from profitable exchange of knowledge and experience.

For this reason, I want to thank pulmonologist friends and colleagues who have shared this path over the years: Giorgio Alcozer, Gianfranco Tassi, Marco Nosenzo, Giampietro Marchetti, Stefano Gasparini, Pier Aldo Canessa, Gian Paolo Ivaldi and others.

But above all, I want to thank a Friend and Colleague with whom I have shared over 30 years of passion for Pleural Pathology: Pier Anselmo Mori. With Anselmo I shared the first experiences in this field, the choice of the most correct tools and methods, and the execution of many thoracoscopies. A special thanks too to my Friend Giampietro Marchetti for his precious contribution to the manual.

Ingredients Needed to Approach Pleural Pathology

- Passion for this important topic: pleural pathology is a patrimony of Pulmonology and all pulmonologists should deal with it personally.
- Not only pneumological skills but also in internal medicine, oncology and infectious disease.
- Ultrasound equipment and the ability to use it.
- Knowledge of the importance, and also the limits, of the study of the pleural fluid.
- Familiarity with all the manoeuvres needed to manage a patient with pleural effusion:
  - thoracic imaging
  - thoracentesis
  - knowledge of the various types of chest drains and how to position them
  - knowledge of the methods of performing pleural biopsy and in particular of Medical Thoracoscopy
- Lots of patience!

Often the diagnosis and management of pleural effusions constitute a challenge requiring various types of medical knowledge, study and dedication—a challenge that unfortunately some pulmonologists decide not to take up, delegating the problem to others (usually thoracic surgeons), thus diminishing the range of our important specialisation.

Special thanks go to Kathleen Ann Jones for her precious help in the creation of the English language version of the Manual.

Her patience and her knowledge of medical English have been of considerable help to me in achieving this aim.

Angelo G. Casalini
Parma, Italy

Introduction

The aim of this book is to be a "Practical Manual".

What does "Practical Manual" mean? And what should a "Practical Manual" be?

Manual:

- A manual is a work that summarises the essential aspects of a specific discipline or topic, generally according to the educational needs of the public to which it is addressed. The term "manual" is the translation of the Greek "encheiridion" (εγχειριδιον), which indicates an object to keep at hand (definition from Wikipedia).
- A book that exposes in a broad and exhaustive way the fundamental news around a given topic (from Treccani encyclopaedia).
- A book that contains the fundamental notions of an art or a discipline, displayed in a way that allows for quick consultation; a book to keep handy (from Garzanti dictionary).

Practical:

- That which is based on direct experience; easily achievable; that which is not lost in abstract matters; that which concerns and serves action (from Garzanti dictionary).

This manual does not claim to address all the topics concerning Pleural Pathology, for which reference should be made to other authoritative texts and to the bibliography that will be reported at the end of each chapter. It is intended to be an easy reference tool for the pulmonologist, the Internist, the General Practitioner, the Thoracic Surgeon and any other doctor dealing with this disease, and an easy and practical reference manual able to provide diagnostic and therapeutic indications for the management of the patient with pleural effusion.

Even if we could do so, we would not wish to simplify such vast and important topics as Clinical Pulmonology and Interventional Pulmonology, but merely to give some "practical" advice to those who are willing to accept it!

Unfortunately, the problems that we often see in the management of pleural effusion are approximate diagnoses, incorrect therapies resulting from superficial diagnoses and unjustified diagnostic and therapeutic delays! One of the biggest problems is precisely the waste of time. "Let's do the thoracentesis and then see ...", "Let's try an antibiotic therapy and then see ...". And the patient waits ... with all that a wait can entail.

Generally, there is little talk of pleural effusion at the various congresses.

In the pneumological environments, we have witnessed in recent years a great and growing interest above all in the development and growth of Interventional Pulmonology, of which the "pleural" methods are an indispensable part and which should be included in the cultural background of the pulmonologist. The widespread use of thoracic ultrasound in the pneumological environment has also played an important role in recent years.

After reading this manual, some zealous readers will perhaps say: "this topic has not been addressed"!

I would like to remind you that this work is neither an encyclopaedia on pleural disease nor a guideline! It is a practical manual, which cannot—and does not aim to—compete with important texts on pleural disease which constitute a rich source of important information and which those who deal with pleural disease know well:

- Jacques Chretien, Jean Bignon, Albert Hirsch. The Pleura in Health and Disease, edited by Jacques Chretien, Dekker New York 1985.
- Giorgio Alcozer. (1984) La toracoscopia diagnostica. Nardini Ed, Firenze.
- Hans-Jürgen Brandt, Robert Loddenkemper, Jutta Mai. Atlas of Diagnostic Thoracoscopy: Indications, Technique. Thieme, 1985.
- Christian Boutin, Jean R Viallat, Yossef Aelony. Practical Thoracoscopy. Springer Verlag. Berlin (1991).
- Angelo G. Casalini. Pneumologia Interventistica. Milano: Springer Italia 2007.
- RW Light, YC Lee, editors. Textbook of Pleural Diseases. 2nd edition. London: Hodder Arnold; 2008.
- Philippe Astoul, GianfrancoTassi, Jean MarieTschopp. Thoracoscopy for Pulmonologists. A Didactic Approach. Berlin, Springer, 2014.
- Richard W Light, YC Gary Lee, editors. Textbook of Pleural Diseases. 3rd edition. 2016 by CRC Press.
- Claudio Sorino, David Feller-Kopman, Giampietro Marchetti. Pleural Diseases. 1st Edition. Clinical Cases and Real World Discussion. Elsevier 2021.

Each chapter of the manual presents diagnostic diagrams, flow charts and practical suggestions on what to do and also what NOT to do since some actions are not useful to the patient or can even be harmful. Each chapter begins with the presentation of one or more clinical cases that are considered explanatory of the path that will be presented later.

These clinical cases are representative of the most frequent clinical situations that pulmonologists or physicians in general have to face in their clinical experience.

There is also an authoritative bibliography to present in greater depth the topics that are of necessity summarised in the text.

Who Is Responsible for Managing Pleural Effusion?

Obviously, those who have the appropriate skills and know-how and are in possession of the necessary diagnostic methods. These skills should be in the possession of the pulmonologist although sometimes this unfortunately does not happen! In many environments, it is easier to entrust the patient to the Thoracic Surgeon and pass on the problems rather than resorting to the methods of Interventional Pulmonology, which require skills, experience and passion. This behaviour causes serious damage and the cultural impoverishment of Pulmonology!

The pulmonologist must have a central role in the management of any pleural effusion of any aetiology and turn to other specialists only when all the tools available to Pulmonology have already been correctly used.

N.B. It is advisable not to store this manual in the library next to little-used books, but to keep it at hand!

Angelo G. Casalini
Parma, Italy

Contents

About the Authors

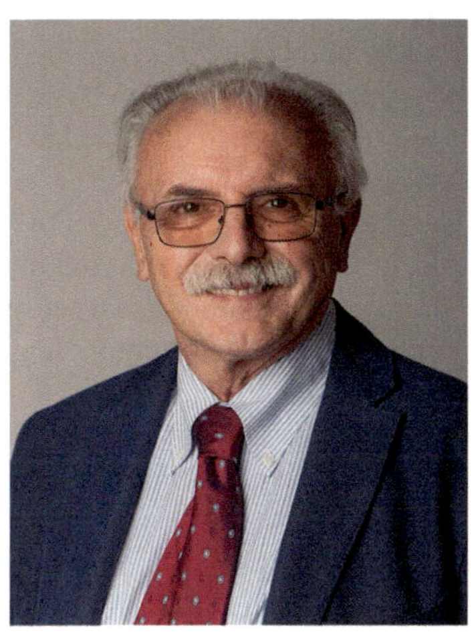

Angelo G. Casalini
is a specialist in Pulmonology and in Hygiene and Preventive Medicine. He worked for over 40 years as a hospital pulmonologist in the Italian public health system. From 2000 to 2002, he was Director of the Pulmonary Department of Cremona Hospital and from 2002 to 2019, he was Director of the Department of Pulmonology and Thoracic Endoscopy of the University Hospital of Parma. He has been an adjunct professor at the School of Specialization in Pulmonology of the University of Milan and at the School of Specialization in Pulmonology of the University of Parma.

His professional activity, in addition to Clinical Pulmonology, has covered all areas of Interventional Pulmonology, in particular Diagnostic Bronchial Endoscopy, Operative Bronchial Endoscopy (with extensive experience in laser therapy and placement of tracheobronchial prostheses), Medical Thoracoscopy (900 Thoracoscopies performed) and Paediatric Bronchial Endoscopy. In addition to his hospital care activities, he has promoted and organised scientific events and congresses and, from 1987 to 2019, he taught 33 theoretical-practical courses in Interventional Pulmonology, aimed at doctors and professional nurses throughout Italy.

This intense teaching activity led to the publication as Editor of the book *Interventional Pulmonology* (Springer), the first Italian text to cover all the methods of Interventional Pulmonology: Diagnostic and Operative Bronchial Endoscopy, Medical Thoracoscopy and Paediatric Bronchial Endoscopy.

He is a member of AIPO (Italian Association of Hospital Pulmonologists), where he was at one time responsible for the scientific area of Interventional Pulmonology and national secretary. He has been a lecturer and invited speaker at numerous national and international courses and congresses.

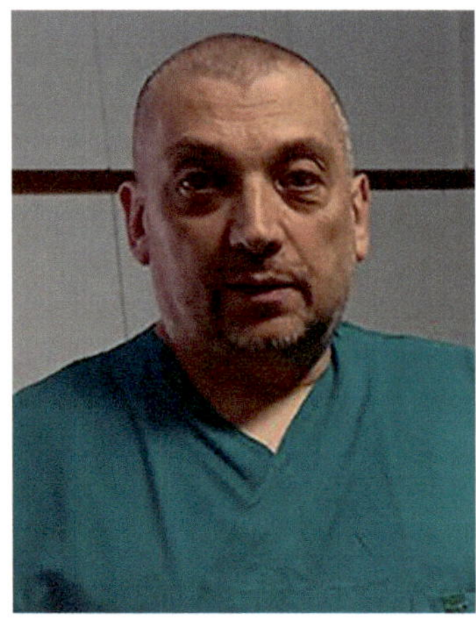

Gian Pietro Marchetti

was born in Brescia (Italy) on June 23, 1961.

In the early years of his clinical activity, he dealt with all sectors of Pulmonology.

He has translated into Italian a Latin book, *Inventum Novum* (1759) by Auenbrugger; he has also published articles on the history of thoracoscopy and on H.C. Jacobaeus, its inventor.

Since 1998, he has worked at the Pulmonology Division of the Spedali Civili in Brescia, where he mainly deals with pleural pathology, while maintaining an active interest in all the issues concerning modern Pulmonology and participating in general daily clinical activity.

He manages a pleural pathology outpatient clinic in this ward, active every day, which treats around 800 patients every year.

He was among the first to use thorax ultrasound, applying it to daily practice and participates every year as a speaker in theoretical-practical courses to Italian pulmonologists.

He has carried out scientific and study activities (more than 100 publications) in an essentially clinical field, with particular reference to pleural pathology, dedicating himself in particular to the development of thoracoscopy and mesothelioma, to thoracic oncology and in general to respiratory diseases.

In 2015, he set up a Facebook group (PLEURAL HUB) where pleural pathology is discussed every day.

He participates as a speaker at numerous national meetings and conferences in the field of thorax ultrasound, pleural pathology and thoracoscopy.

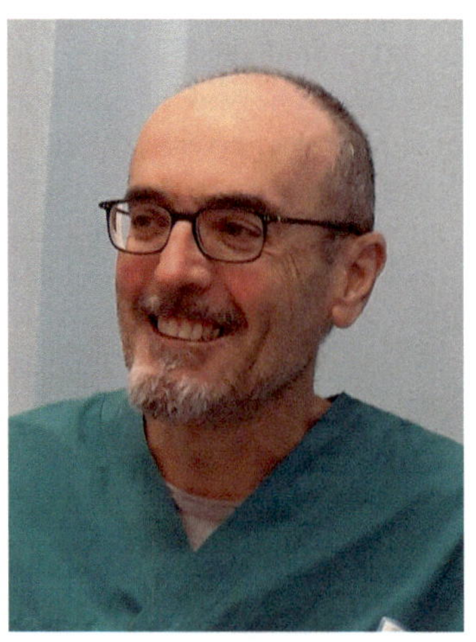

Pier Anselmo Mori

was born in Parma (Italy) on August 24, 1957.

He holds a specialisation in Pulmonology; he worked as a pulmonologist in the Unit of Pulmonology and Thoracic Endoscopy of the University Hospital of Parma from June 1989 to August 2022.

His professional activity, besides that of "Clinical Pulmonology", was dedicated to tuberculosis and infectious diseases and pleural pathology, i.e. the understanding of ultrasound, thoracentesis, pleural drainage and medical thoracoscopy.

In addition to his hospital clinical activity, he was regularly invited as a speaker to various scientific events and congresses.

His medical and scientific activity has led to several publications in medical journals.

He was an adjunct professor at the School of Specialisation in Pulmonology of the University of Parma.

He is a member of AIPO, of which he is among those responsible for the scientific area of Infectious Pulmonary Diseases and is a former president of the Emilia-Romagna regional section.

Clinical-Instrumental Diagnostic Approach to Pleural Effusion

Content

Clinical-Instrumental Diagnostic Approach to Pleural Effusion

Preliminary Clinical and Laboratory Evaluation Common to All Patients

Angelo G. Casalini

Contents

A. G. Casalini (ed.), *Practical Manual of Pleural Pathology*,
https://doi.org/10.1007/978-3-031-20312-1_1

1

About 15–20% of hospitalisations present in Pneumology are pleural diseases

Pleural diseases account for about 15–20% of hospitalisations in the pulmonology units; the correct management of the patient with pleural effusion requires specific pulmonological skills and more, in order to establish a correct diagnostic approach each time [1–4] based on the clinical presentation, thus taking into account the clinical manifestations and the consequent diagnostic hypotheses; it is important to avoid useless and unmotivated therapies, which unfortunately are still undertaken without any logic, entailing negative diagnostic delays for the patient.

The guidelines of the BTS [3] also recognise the pulmonologist's skills and means for the correct management of pleural effusion.

Most frequent causes: heart failure, infectious effusions (including tuberculosis), neoplastic effusions, pulmonary embolism

The causes of pleural effusion are numerous (◘ Table 1.1) [5], and many of those listed in the table are actually very rare. The most frequent – and those with which we are confronted

◘ Table 1.1 Causes of pleural effusion

Causes of pleural effusion	
Exudates	**Transudates**
Infectious • Parapneumonic • Empyema • Tuberculosis • Viral • Other	Congestive heart failure
Neoplastic: • Metastatic effusion • Mesothelioma	Hepatic hydrothorax
Paramalignant effusion	Nephrotic syndrome
Pulmonary embolism	Pulmonary embolism
Abdominal diseases	Peritoneal dialysis
Cardiac diseases or problems	Hypoalbuminaemia
Gynaecological diseases	Atelectasis
Collagen vascular diseases	Superior vena cava obstruction
Drugs	Trapped lung
Haemothorax	Sarcoidosis
Chylothorax	Myxedema
Sarcoidosis	Urinothorax
Miscellaneous	Pulmonary arterial hypertension
	Glomerulonephritis
	Pericardial disease

daily in pneumological practice – are heart failure effusion, infectious effusions including tuberculosis, neoplastic effusions and pulmonary embolism. It is important to know the wide and often complex field of causes in order to be able to competently face the difficult aspect of differential diagnosis.

The diagnosis of pleural effusion is generally easy and can also be made simply with a correct physical examination of the patient and confirmed by a simple chest X-ray or by an ultrasound check; the aetiological diagnosis, on the other hand, is often complex, requiring specific skills, the availability of suitable tools and the implementation of dedicated diagnostic paths; this is what this manual proposes to elucidate.

1.1 Clinical Onset

Clinical manifestations often allow for a diagnostic orientation

The symptoms that accompany the clinical onset of pleural effusion can very often already be indicative, allowing for diagnostic hypotheses, which, however, will later have to be validated with further investigations [3].

In particular, the presence or absence of fever is an excellent element that allows us with good precision to distinguish pleural effusions with an infectious aetiology from those with another aetiology [6]. This element is of fundamental importance, as in the presence of an infectious effusion the clinical approach necessarily requires a tight time frame in order to distinguish complicated parapneumonic effusions and empyema from others in the context of infectious aetiology effusions and to establish a correct and prompt treatment, for which reference should be made to the dedicated chapter.

The onset symptomatology can be modest and subtle, with gradual onset, the only symptom being progressively worsening dyspnoea. In some situations, the symptoms may be more marked with acute onset of severe dyspnoea (never forget that pulmonary embolism is the 4th cause of pleural effusion!). It may be accompanied by typical chest pain related to deep inspiration or atypical pain, or cough, usually dry. Symptoms may be related to the underlying disease that caused the effusion, such as haemoptysis in the case of lung cancer, or mucopurulent sputum in the case of parapneumonic effusion.

Pleural effusion from heart failure is the most frequent cause; importance of the clinical presentation!

The appearance of bilateral pleural effusion accompanied by dyspnoea requires a rapid and correct cardiac evaluation of the patient, as in many cases it can already be indicative for a diagnosis of heart failure effusion (the first cause of pleural effusion).

The patient's medical history must also be investigated for existing or pre-existing neoplastic and non-neoplastic diseases (e.g. connective tissue diseases), occupational exposure and the possible intake of drugs that can cause pleural effusion [7] (nitrofurantoin, dantrolene, methysergide, amiodarone, interleukin-2, procarbazine, methotrexate, clozapine, phenytoin, beta-blockers and others); there are few pleural effusions caused by drugs but it is important to think about this aetiology especially in the case of eosinophilic effusion in which another aetiology is not recognised. In case of clinical doubt, please refer to the ► pneumotox.com website.

The questions to ask when faced with a patient with pleural effusion are the following:

- which symptoms are really important and possibly indicative of a diagnostic hypothesis?
- what is the role of imaging (chest X-ray, ultrasound, CT, PET)?
- what tests should we ask the laboratory to perform on blood samples and on the fluid taken with thoracentesis?
- what are the limits of clinical diagnosis and non-invasive or limited invasive methods?
- when and why is it necessary to resort to invasive investigations and which methods should we choose?

The initial approach therefore includes a detailed medical history, a complete objective examination and a chest X-ray. At this point, it is often possible to make diagnostic hypotheses. However, it is necessary to follow a diagnostic path common to all pleural effusions; the one represented in the flow chart below (◘ Fig. 1.1) can be of great use.

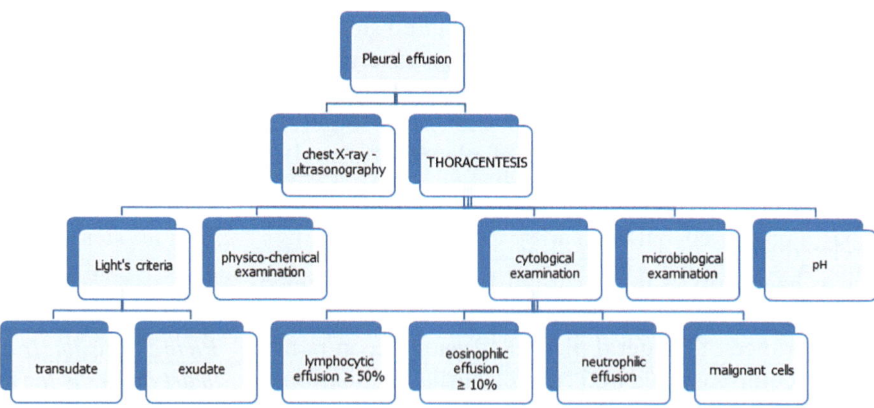

◘ **Fig. 1.1** Basic diagnostic path to follow for all patients with pleural effusion

1.2 Radiological Investigations

Ultrasound is essential for the characteristics of the effusion and as a guide to thoracentesis

Chest X-ray (necessarily performed in 2 projections) is the first fundamental radiological investigation and yields important information about the effusion: location, extent, possible bilaterality. Ultrasound evaluation is the most important integration of chest X-ray and provides us with additional important information about the effusion: characteristics of the fluid, presence or absence of any loculated collections; it is also an important guide in choosing the best place to perform an exploratory puncture or place a drain. The next investigation is the chest CT scan, the usefulness of which, in particular in neoplastic and infectious effusions, will be evaluated in detail in the next chapters.

1.3 Thoracentesis

Thoracentesis must always be performed within 24–48 h

Thoracentesis is the fundamental diagnostic investigation, which, however, is often not performed in the correct time, or else not all the necessary investigations on the pleural fluid are performed; the only situation in which it is not necessary to perform all the investigations is when a diagnosis already exists and thoracentesis is performed only for evacuation purposes; unfortunately, in some situations, repeated and useless thoracenteses are performed in the hope of obtaining a diagnosis, and this leads to unjustified diagnostic delays; a delayed aetiological diagnosis may be associated with increased morbidity and mortality.

Virtually all patients with pleural effusions should undergo thoracentesis, except in cases of haemodynamic pleural effusion (some clarifications will be made in the dedicated chapter) and very modest pleural effusions (<1 cm); however, modest pleural effusions must be carefully monitored as there may be a rapid increase in the effusion even in the following 24 h, entailing the need to intervene.

The use of thoracic ultrasound is considered almost indispensable for the execution of thoracentesis as it minimises the risks of complications [8], in particular of perforation of the lung and vessels, and improves the recovery of pleural fluid, enabling access even to slight and loculated collections.

1.4 Pleural Fluid Examination

Always include the differential cell count in the investigations to be performed on the pleural fluid

Once the pleural fluid has been obtained, it is necessary to perform all laboratory investigations [9], which include: physico-chemical examination, complete microbiological examination (specific requests based on clinical doubt), cytological examination, differential cell count (especially essential in effusions in which an infectious aetiology is suspected) and pH, performed with a blood gas analyser [10]. The presence of a lymphocytic effusion, for example, can be indicative of various diseases or situations: tuberculous pleurisy, chylothorax, lymphoma, yellow nail syndrome, rheumatoid arthritis, sarcoidosis or post aortocoronary bypass [11]. The use of Light's criteria [12] is important to distinguish exudative effusions from transudates; see the chapter dedicated to transudatory effusions. The pleural fluid present in physiological conditions is a transudate and is transformed into an exudate in pathological situations. An effusion is defined as exudative when at least one of the following criteria is present:

- ratio between pleural fluid proteins and serum proteins >0.5
- ratio between LDH in pleural fluid and LDH in serum >0.6
- LDH of pleural fluid >2/3 of the upper limit of the normal level of LDH in serum

Through Light's criteria, it is possible, with excellent approximation, to distinguish transudates from exudates and hence to obtain an initial diagnostic orientation. Other investigations can be used in doubtful cases; see the chapter on transudative pleural effusion.

Therefore, the complete evaluation of the pleural fluid [13] should always include:

(a) macroscopic characteristics of the pleural fluid: haematic, purulent, cloudy, etc.;
(b) odour: anaerobic infection;
(c) the distinction between exudate and transudate;
(d) the differential cell count;
(e) the search for neoplastic cells;
(f) the complete microbiological examination;
(g) the pH;
(h) glucose;
(i) amylase.

The differential cell count, which plays an important role and provides a useful diagnostic orientation in particular in infectious effusions, is unfortunately not performed routinely; the topic will be explored in depth in the chapter on infectious effusions.

It is important to remember that the causes of a pleural effusion can be more than one at the same time. In this study [14], in 30% of cases, the cause of the effusion was multifactorial. It is important to remember this possibility in particular in cardiopathic patients, because of the possible concomitance of other diseases associated with heart failure.

The evaluation of the clinical data associated with the results of the complete investigations of the pleural fluid leads to a diagnosis in about 75% of pleural effusions [15, 16] (◘ Table 1.2).

In the remaining 25% of patients, it is necessary to investigate further; this requires a biopsy of the pleura, usually thoracoscopically.

In 25% of patients with pleural effusion, a pleural biopsy is required

◘ **Table 1.2** From Sahn [15]

Disease	Pleural fluid analysis
Empyema	Observation of the pleural fluid; culture
Malignancy	Positive cytology
Lupus pleurisy	LE cells present
Tuberculous effusion	Microbiology
Oesophageal rupture	High amylase, pleural fluid acidosis
Fungal pleurisy	Microbiology
Chylothorax	Triglycerides (>110 mg/dL); lipoprotein electrophoresis (chylomicrons)
Haemothorax	Haematocrit (pleural fluid/blood ratio >0.5)
Urinothorax	Creatinine (pleural fluid/serum ratio >1.0)
Peritoneal dialysis	Protein (<1 g/dL) glucose (300–400 mg/dL)
Extravascular migration of a central venous catheter	Observation (milky if lipids are infused); glucose PF/serum >1.0
Rheumatoid pleurisy	Characteristic cytology

1

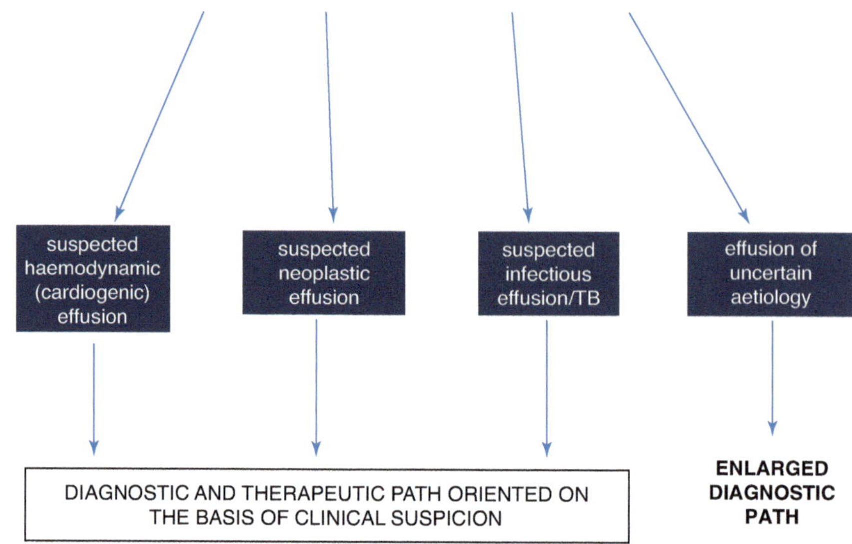

Fig. 1.2 Insights following clinical suspicion

The diagnostic and therapeutic process continues on the basis of the initial clinical orientation and must be integrated with more targeted investigations (Fig. 1.2) and dedicated paths, which will be presented and explained in the next chapters.

References

1. McGrath EE, Anderson PB. Diagnosis of pleural effusion: a systematic approach. Am J Crit Care. 2011;20(2):119–27; quiz 128. https://doi.org/10.4037/ajcc2011685. PMID: 21362716.
2. Aboudara M, Maldonado F. Update in the management of pleural effusions. Med Clin North Am. 2019;103(3):475–85. https://doi.org/10.1016/j.mcna.2018.12.007. PMID: 30955515.
3. Hooper C, Lee YC, Maskell N, BTS Pleural Guideline Group. Investigation of a unilateral pleural effusion in adults: British Thoracic Society Pleural Disease Guideline 2010. Thorax. 2010;65(Suppl 2):4–17. https://doi.org/10.1136/thx.2010.136978. PMID: 20696692.
4. Rahman NM, Chapman SJ, Davies RJ. Pleural effusion: a structured approach to care. Br Med Bull. 2005;72:31–47. https://doi.org/10.1093/bmb/ldh040. PMID: 15767562.
5. Feller-Kopman D, Light R. Pleural disease. N Engl J Med. 2018;378(8):740–51. https://doi.org/10.1056/NEJMra1403503. PMID: 29466146.
6. Bhatnagar R, Maskell N. The modern diagnosis and management of pleural effusions. BMJ. 2015;351:h4520. https://doi.org/10.1136/bmj.h4520. PMID: 26350935.

7. Huggins JT, Sahn SA. Drug-induced pleural disease. Clin Chest Med. 2004;25(1):141–53. https://doi.org/10.1016/S0272-5231(03)00125-4. PMID: 15062606.
8. Wrightson JM, Fysh E, Maskell NA, Lee YC. Risk reduction in pleural procedures: sonography, simulation and supervision. Curr Opin Pulm Med. 2010;16(4):340–50. https://doi.org/10.1097/MCP.0b013e32833a233b. PMID: 20531083.
9. Sahn SA. The value of pleural fluid analysis. Am J Med Sci. 2008;335(1):7–15. https://doi.org/10.1097/MAJ.0b013e31815d25e6. PMID: 18195577.
10. Cheng DS, Rodriguez RM, Rogers J, Wagster M, Starnes DL, Light RW. Comparison of pleural fluid pH values obtained using blood gas machine, pH meter, and pH indicator strip. Chest. 1998;114(5):1368–72. https://doi.org/10.1378/chest.114.5.1368. PMID: 9824016.
11. Sahn SA. Pleural disease. In: ACCP pulmonary medicine board review. 25th ed. Glenview: ACCP; 2009. p. 513–46.
12. Light RW, Macgregor MI, Luchsinger PC, Ball WC Jr. Pleural effusions: the diagnostic separation of transudates and exudates. Ann Intern Med. 1972;77(4):507–13. https://doi.org/10.7326/0003-4819-77-4-507. PMID: 4642731.
13. Zuccatosta L. Il versamento pleurico: aspetti eziologici, diagnostici e clinici. In: Casalini AG, editor. Pneumologia Interventistica. Milano: Springer Italia; 2007.
14. Bintcliffe OJ, Hooper CE, Rider IJ, Finn RS, Morley AJ, Zahan-Evans N, Harvey JE, Skyrme-Jones AP, Maskell NA. Unilateral pleural effusions with more than one apparent etiology. A prospective observational study. Ann Am Thorac Soc. 2016;13(7):1050–6. https://doi.org/10.1513/AnnalsATS.201601-082OC. PMID: 27064965.
15. Sahn SA. The diagnostic value of pleural fluid analysis. Semin Respir Crit Care Med. 1995;16:269–78. https://doi.org/10.1055/s-2007-1009837.
16. Jany B, Welte T. Pleural effusion in adults-etiology, diagnosis, and treatment. Dtsch Arztebl Int. 2019;116(21):377–86. https://doi.org/10.3238/arztebl.2019.0377. PMID: 31315808; PMCID: PMC6647819.

Transudative Pleural Effusion

Content

Transudative Pleural Effusion

Angelo G. Casalini

Contents

A. G. Casalini (ed.), *Practical Manual of Pleural Pathology*,
https://doi.org/10.1007/978-3-031-20312-1_2

2

The distinction between transudate and exudate should always be a starting point in the evaluation of a patient with pleural effusion, but unfortunately it is not always taken into consideration. Many times I have asked medical students or even recent graduates who attended the ward: how is a transudate distinguished from an exudate? I had the strangest answers: from the colour (if it is clear it is a transudate), from the specific weight etc. Very few answered correctly the question: do you know what Light's criteria are and what they are for?

Importance of Light's criteria, neglected or misinterpreted

The distinction between transudate and exudate is of fundamental importance as the diagnostic, prognostic and therapeutic implications of a transudate are completely different from those of an exudate. Light's criteria [1], although not infallible, are certainly very indicative; although other investigations over time have been proposed for this purpose, they remain a fundamental step in the evaluation of a pleural effusion. The limitation of Light's criteria is that they can identify 15–20% of transudates as exudates as they have a very high sensitivity (98%) but a lower specificity (83%).

A pleural fluid is defined as exudate [1] when at least one of the following characteristics is present: ratio between total proteins in the pleural fluid and total proteins in serum >0.5; ratio between LDH in pleural fluid and LDH in serum >0.6; level of LDH in the pleural fluid >2/3 of the normal upper limit of LDH in the blood [2]. Other criteria have been proposed for pleural effusions suspected of being related to heart failure, but with Light's criteria showing an exudate; they are generally used infrequently, because they are little known, but they can be very important in doubtful cases. One of these is the measurement of the albumin concentration gradient between serum and pleural fluid. In almost all patients with transudative effusion, this gradient exceeds 1.2 mg/dL. Another criterion is the concentration of cholesterol in the pleural fluid >60 mg/dL. For further information, see the scientific literature [3–5]. Like all laboratory tests, Light's criteria must also be used with 'prudence', because of their possible limits.

The most frequent cause of transudate: heart failure; the clinical presentation is fundamental

The most frequent cause of pleural effusion is heart failure [6]; this datum is also confirmed in other experiences [7]. Other cases, however, yielded different results; Porcel [8], for example, in a series of 3077 patients recorded heart failure in second place (21%), with neoplastic effusion in first place (27%).

Sometimes the clinical signs and symptoms are already strongly indicative as there are previous anamnestic data, orthopnoea, paroxysmal nocturnal dyspnoea, peripheral oedema or the presence of chest X-ray cardiomegaly; often it is not enough that the patient is cardiopathic to consider the effusion on a cardiogenic basis; the possibility should be considered that a cardiopathic patient could have a pleural effusion of another nature [9].

In the heart patient, carefully evaluate an exudative effusion ...

Although heart failure produces transudative effusion, some authors [10] found that about half of patients with a clinical diagnosis of heart failure had exudative effusion according to Light's criteria. Associated diseases were present in most cases, but in about 1/3 of the exudates, the cause was related to heart failure. For this reason, the diagnostic approach often has to be integrated [11]. If it is a transudate, the therapy indicated for heart failure is established; if it is an exudate, other investigations are necessary, such as measuring the albumin concentration gradient between serum and pleural fluid. It must be taken into account that an 'acute' diuretic treatment (e.g. furosemide IV) can convert a transudate into an exudate [12]; this conversion from transudate to exudate following diuretic therapy is confirmed by many authors [13]. It is also important to remember that the causes of a pleural effusion can be more than one at the same time; in Bintcliffe's study [14], in 30% of cases, the cause of the effusion was multifactorial.

The following flow chart (◘ Fig. 2.1) can be indicative of a correct diagnostic and therapeutic approach in the presence of pleural effusion in a patient with signs and symptoms of heart failure. It is important to underline that, if the patient is heavily dyspnoeic and the effusion is abundant, without waiting for the response to diuretic therapy we need to perform an evacuative thoracentesis or place a small-bore drain (such as a pig tail), to allow the patient to resume breathing! Another aspect to remember is that flow charts are not infallible and must always be discussed and followed critically!

Other possible and relatively frequent causes of transudate:
- *hepatic hydrothorax*
- *peritoneal dialysis*
- *nephrotic syndrome*
- *pulmonary embolism*

In common practice, the vast majority of transudates are caused by heart failure, followed by cirrhosis of the liver (hepatic hydrothorax) [15]; in pulmonary embolism, the effusion can be an exudate or a transudate; according to Light, pulmonary embolism is the 4th cause of pleural effusions after heart failure, infections and neoplasms!

Hepatic hydrothorax is defined as the presence of pleural effusion in a patient with liver cirrhosis and portal hypertension without concomitant cardiac, pulmonary or pleural diseases. It is found in about 5% to 10% of patients with liver cirrhosis, and in around 80% of these, it is concomitant with ascites [16]. In 18% of cases of hepatic hydrothorax, the effusion can appear as an exudate [3].

Other causes of transudative effusion can be peritoneal dialysis [17], nephrotic syndrome [18], obstruction of the supe-

pleural effusion from suspected heart failure
-Chest X-ray
-ultrasound
modest bilateral effusion
indicated therapy (diuretics)
Light's criteria
transudate
indicated cardiological therapy (diuretics)
exudate?
serum/pleural fluid albumin concentration gradient
> di 1.2 mg/dl
most likely transudate
if effusion is important, carry out evacuative thoracentesis
indicated cardiological therapy (diuretics) and observation
< di 1.2.mg/dl
exudate
widen the investigation
Light's criteria:
- pleural fluid proteins/serum proteins > 0.5
- pleural fluid LDH/serum LDH> 0.6
- pleural fluid LDH > 200 IU or> 2/3 upper
limit LDH in serum

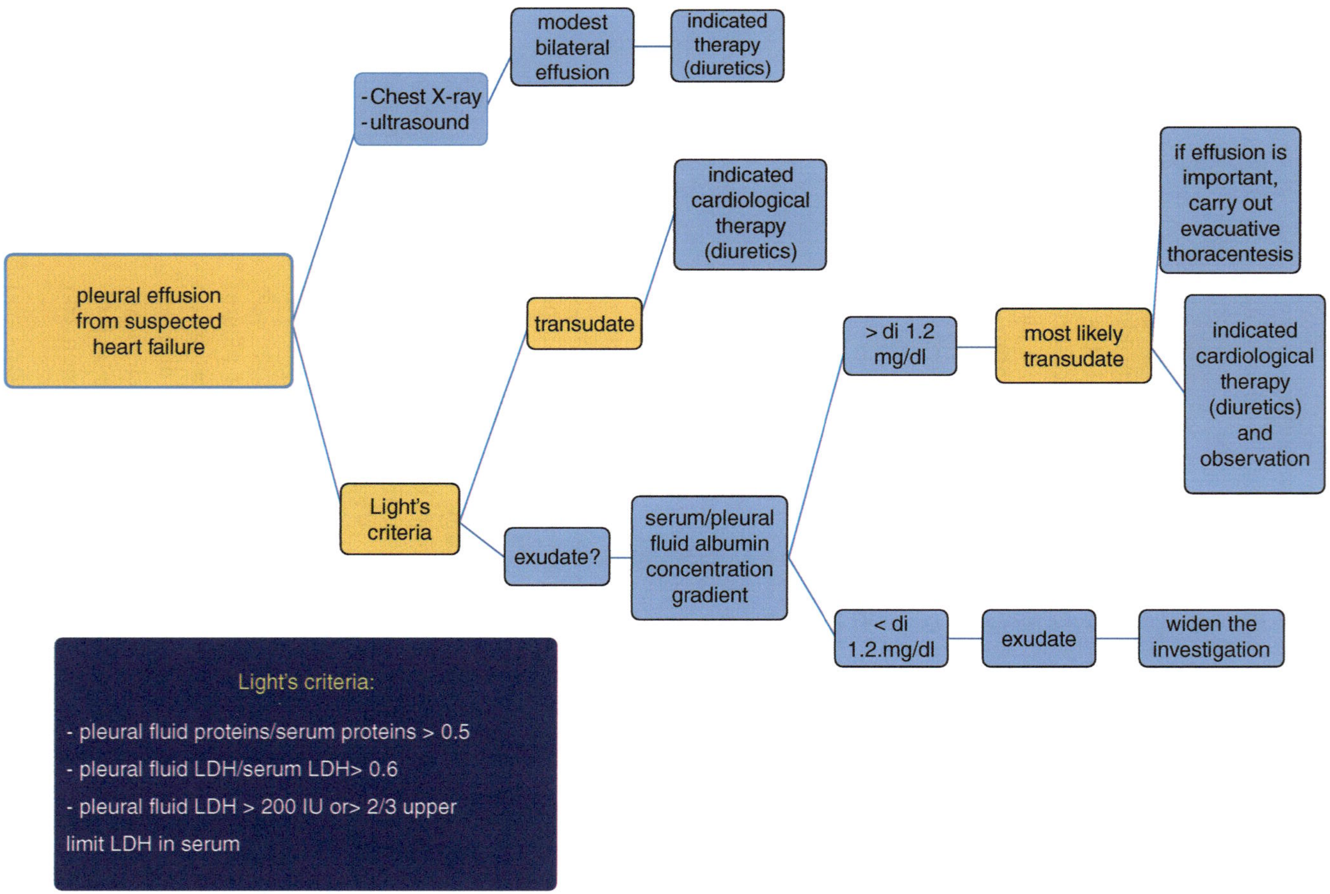

Fig. 2.1 Diagnostic-therapeutic approach for patients with heart failure and pleural effusion

rior vena cava and hypoalbuminaemia. The presence of these effusions, although benign, has an important prognostic implication. In this large study [19] of non-neoplastic pleural effusions secondary to heart, liver or kidney failure, the prognosis was poor with a high 1-year mortality, of 57%, 46% and 25%, respectively.

References

1. Light RW, Macgregor MI, Luchsinger PC, Ball WC Jr. Pleural effusions: the diagnostic separation of transudates and exudates. Ann Intern Med. 1972;77(4):507–13. https://doi.org/10.7326/0003-4819-77-4-507. PMID: 4642731.
2. Light RW. Diagnostic principles in pleural disease. Eur Respir J. 1997;10(2):476–81. https://doi.org/10.1183/09031936.97.10020476. PMID: 9042652.
3. Bielsa S, Porcel JM, Castellote J, Mas E, Esquerda A, Light RW. Solving the Light's criteria misclassification rate of cardiac and hepatic transudates. Respirology. 2012;17(4):721–6. https://doi.org/10.1111/j.1440-1843.2012.02155.x. PMID: 22372660.
4. Han ZJ, Wu XD, Cheng JJ, Zhao SD, Gao MZ, Huang HY, Gu B, Ma P, Chen Y, Wang JH, Yang CJ, Yan ZH. Diagnostic accuracy of natriuretic peptides for heart failure in patients with pleural effusion: a systematic review and updated meta-analysis. PLoS One. 2015;10(8):e0134376. https://doi.org/10.1371/journal.pone.0134376. PMID: 26244664; PMCID: PMC4526570.
5. Porcel JM. Identifying transudates misclassified by Light's criteria. Curr Opin Pulm Med. 2013;19(4):362–7. https://doi.org/10.1097/MCP.0b013e32836022dc. PMID: 23508114.
6. Light RW. Pleural effusions. Med Clin North Am. 2011;95(6):1055–70. https://doi.org/10.1016/j.mcna.2011.08.005. Epub 2011 Sep 25. PMID: 22032427.
7. Korczyński P, Górska K, Konopka D, Al-Haj D, Filipiak KJ, Krenke R. Significance of congestive heart failure as a cause of pleural effusion: pilot data from a large multidisciplinary teaching hospital. Cardiol J. 2020;27(3):254–61. https://doi.org/10.5603/CJ.a2018.0137. Epub 2018 Nov 8. PMID: 30406935; PMCID: PMC8015984.
8. Porcel JM, Esquerda A, Vives M, Bielsa S. Etiology of pleural effusions: analysis of more than 3,000 consecutive thoracenteses. Arch Bronconeumol. 2014;50(5):161–5. https://doi.org/10.1016/j.arbres.2013.11.007. Epub 2013 Dec 20. PMID: 24360987.
9. Gotsman I, Fridlender Z, Meirovitz A, Dratva D, Muszkat M. The evaluation of pleural effusions in patients with heart failure. Am J Med. 2001;111(5):375–8. https://doi.org/10.1016/s0002-9343(01)00881-6. PMID: 11583640.
10. Eid AA, Keddissi JI, Samaha M, Tawk MM, Kimmell K, Kinasewitz GT. Exudative effusions in congestive heart failure. Chest. 2002;122(5):1518–23. https://doi.org/10.1378/chest.122.5.1518. PMID: 12426246.
11. Mitrouska I, Bouros D. The trans-exudative pleural effusion. Chest. 2002;122(5):1503–5. https://doi.org/10.1378/chest.122.5.1503. PMID: 12426239.

2

12. Chakko SC, Caldwell SH, Sforza PP. Treatment of congestive heart failure. Its effect on pleural fluid chemistry. Chest. 1989;95(4):798–802. https://doi.org/10.1378/chest.95.4.798. PMID: 2924609.
13. Romero-Candeira S, Fernández C, Martín C, Sánchez-Paya J, Hernández L. Influence of diuretics on the concentration of proteins and other components of pleural transudates in patients with heart failure. Am J Med. 2001;110(9):681–6. https://doi.org/10.1016/s0002-9343(01)00726-4. PMID: 11403751.
14. Bintcliffe OJ, Hooper CE, Rider IJ, Finn RS, Morley AJ, Zahan-Evans N, Harvey JE, Skyrme-Jones AP, Maskell NA. Unilateral pleural effusions with more than one apparent etiology. A prospective observational study. Ann Am Thorac Soc. 2016;13(7):1050–6. https://doi.org/10.1513/AnnalsATS.201601-082OC. PMID: 27064965.
15. Ferreiro L, Porcel JM, Valdés L. Diagnosis and management of pleural transudates. Arch Bronconeumol. 2017;53(11):629–36. https://doi.org/10.1016/j.arbres.2017.04.018. Epub 2017 Jun 19. PMID: 28641878.
16. Porcel JM. Management of refractory hepatic hydrothorax. Curr Opin Pulm Med. 2014;20(4):352–7. https://doi.org/10.1097/MCP.0000000000000058. PMID: 24811830.
17. Nomoto Y, Suga T, Nakajima K, Sakai H, Osawa G, Ota K, Kawaguchi Y, Sakai T, Sakai S, Shibata M, et al. Acute hydrothorax in continuous ambulatory peritoneal dialysis–a collaborative study of 161 centers. Am J Nephrol. 1989;9(5):363–7. https://doi.org/10.1159/000167997. PMID: 2679094.
18. Light RW. The undiagnosed pleural effusion. Clin Chest Med. 2006;27(2):309–19. https://doi.org/10.1016/j.ccm.2005.12.002. PMID: 16716820.
19. Walker SP, Morley AJ, Stadon L, De Fonseka D, Arnold DT, Medford ARL, Maskell NA. Nonmalignant pleural effusions: a prospective study of 356 consecutive unselected patients. Chest. 2017;151(5):1099–105. https://doi.org/10.1016/j.chest.2016.12.014. Epub 2016 Dec 23. PMID: 28025056.

Exudative Pleural Effusions: Primary Neoplastic Pleural Effusion

Contents

Clinical Case of Malignant Pleural Mesothelioma

Angelo G. Casalini

Contents

A. G. Casalini (ed.), *Practical Manual of Pleural Pathology*,
https://doi.org/10.1007/978-3-031-20312-1_3

We here report the case of a 79-year-old patient, an entrepreneur with no occupational exposure to asbestos, a non-smoker with no serious diseases in his medical history except hiatal hernia with GE reflux. His general condition was excellent; until a few weeks before admission, he played tennis regularly. Subsequently, there was an increasingly limiting dyspnoea from exertion, and a dry cough, but never fever.

On physical examination of the chest, there were signs of left pleural effusion; chest X-ray was performed (◘ Fig. 3.1), confirming the presence of a left pleural effusion. There was nothing relevant to report in haematological tests.

The clinical onset without fever, in the absence of previous diseases and only with progressive dyspnoea, may already be indicative of a neoplastic effusion, and therefore, we decided to perform a Medical Thoracoscopy immediately instead of performing a thoracentesis and waiting for the results of the pleural fluid tests (about 6 days for the cytological test!), which are diagnostic in around 60% of neoplastic effusions and in 30% of mesotheliomas. Medical thoracoscopy was carried out in the endoscopy suite; the patient lay on his healthy side under local anaesthesia with 2% lidocaine and moderate sedation using midazolam, according to the technique described by Boutin [1] using a rigid 7-mm trocar (Wolf). The instrument was introduced in the left anterior axillary line, after ultrasound examination.

The pleural cavity contained numerous fibrin adhesions which were partially removed with the forceps; approximately 600 ml of bloody pleural fluid were aspirated. The parietal pleura was considerably and diffusely thickened, with rare

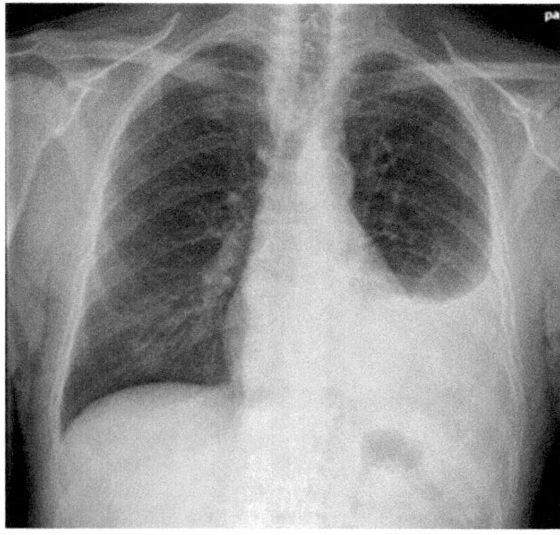

◘ **Fig. 3.1** Chest X-ray at admission

nodules of differing dimension: the macroscopic appearance was strongly indicative of neoplasia (◘ Fig. 3.2).

Repeated biopsies were performed, and at the end of the examination, talc poudrage was performed (4 g of Steritalc-Novatech) followed by the positioning of pleural drainage in suction. At the radiological check-up after 5 days (◘ Fig. 3.3), only obliteration of the sinus remained, with no more fluid from the drainage; the drain was removed and the patient was discharged.

The biopsies enabled the histological diagnosis of desmoplastic sarcomatoid mesothelioma, and the cytological examination was negative. In agreement with the oncologist, it was

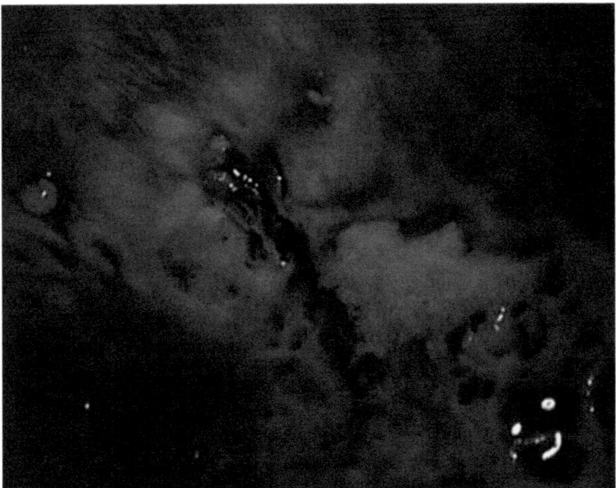

◘ **Fig. 3.2** Endoscopic picture

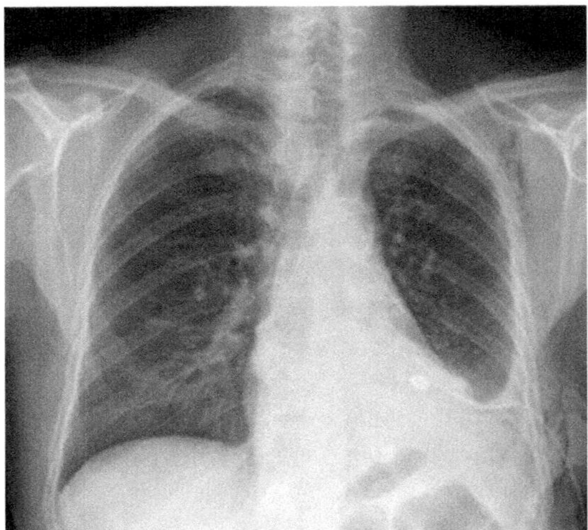

◘ **Fig. 3.3** Chest X-ray after 5 days

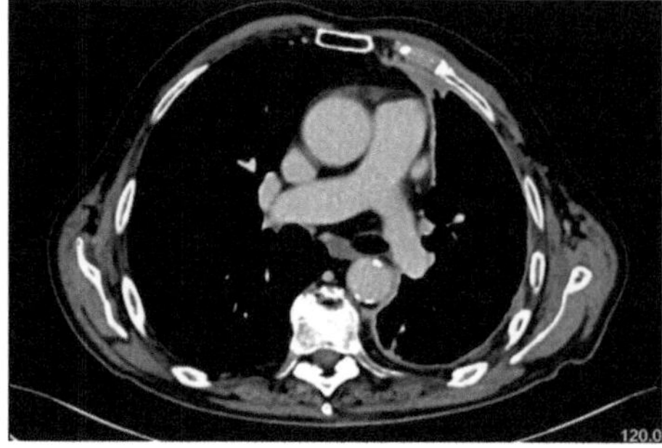

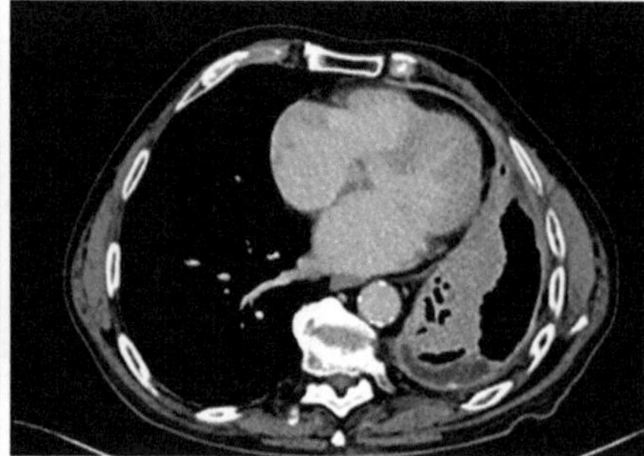

Fig. 3.4 CT 1 year after diagnosis

decided not to proceed with chemotherapy, but only with a clinical follow-up. We had previously published our experience of a small series of patients with desmoplastic mesothelioma [2]. According to the 2010 Guidelines of the European Respiratory Society (ERS) and the European Society of Thoracic Surgeons (ESTS) [3], desmoplastic MPM is considered a variant of sarcomatous MPM, in which at least 50% of the tumour mass is made up of dense paucicellular connective tissue and sarcomatous foci of cells arranged in lamellar spaces in a disorganised way with sometimes atypical nuclei. The prognosis is poor and characterised by an often rapid clinical course with metastasis in 30% of cases in the liver, lungs, kidneys and bones. A careful medical investigation did not establish any occupational or environmental exposure to asbestos in our patient.

At the CT after 12 months, the presence of the typical 'pleural rind' and the complete absence of pleural fluid were documented (Fig. 3.4).

The patient passed away 14 months after diagnosis.

Conclusive Comments

The clinical case presented may provoke comments on the diagnostic-therapeutic strategy followed.

Most likely in other medical settings, the diagnostic path would have been different and would certainly have started with a diagnostic thoracentesis.

The two most important objectives in situations like the one presented are:

1. to reach a definite diagnosis
2. to solve the problem of the recurrence of the pleural effusion and the related dyspnoea.

The immediate diagnostic approach directly with Medical Thoracoscopy allowed us in only a week to achieve both these results!

See the Flow chart in the chapter on Malignant Pleural Mesothelioma and in the chapter on Secondary neoplastic pleural effusion.

References

1. Boutin C, Viallat JR, Aelony Y. Practical thoracoscopy. Berlin: Springer Verlag; 1991.
2. Casalini AG, Mori PA, Melioli A, Rindi G, Lasagna L, Sabbadini F, Tafuro F, Bertorelli G. Mesotelioma maligno desmoplastico: presentazione di 4 casi clinici e breve revisione della letteratura. Desmoplastic malignant mesothelioma: 4 clinical cases and review of the literature. Rassegna Patol dell'Apparato Resp. 2011;26:18–23.
3. Scherpereel A, Astoul P, Baas P, Berghmans T, Clayson H, de Vuyst P, Dienemann H, Galateau-Salle F, Hennequin C, Hillerdal G, Le Péchoux C, Mutti L, Pairon JC, Stahel R, van Houtte P, van Meerbeeck J, Waller D, Weder W. European Respiratory Society/European Society of Thoracic Surgeons Task Force. Guidelines of the European Respiratory Society and the European Society of Thoracic Surgeons for the management of malignant pleural mesothelioma. Eur Respir J. 2010;35(3):479–95. https://doi.org/10.1183/09031936.00063109. Epub 2009 Aug 28. PMID: 19717482.

Malignant Pleural Mesothelioma

Angelo G. Casalini

Contents

A. G. Casalini (ed.), *Practical Manual of Pleural Pathology*,
https://doi.org/10.1007/978-3-031-20312-1_4

In Italy, about 1500 mesotheliomas are diagnosed per year compared to over 35,000 lung cancers

The current reality in Italy regarding Malignant Pleural Mesothelioma (MPM) [1] according to the data provided by the Italian Register of Malignant Mesothelioma (ReNaM) in 2018 [2] is the following: incidence of 3.26 cases per 100,000 inhabitants/year in men and 0.86 in women. In Italy, the median survival [3] in the period 1990–2001 was 9.8 months, with a 3-year survival of less than 10%. The incidence of MPM differs at regional level because of environmental problems and occupational exposure; in recent years it seems to be stabilising at around 1500 cases/year at national level, pending a hoped for decline. No type of treatment is associated with a statistical improvement in survival. From this, we deduce the great importance that 'palliative' type interventions can have, aimed at improving the quality of life (see clinical case presented!).

In most cases, the patient with MPM pleural effusion is hospitalised in Pneumology, or the intervention of the Pulmonologist is in any case requested. The first goal we set ourselves is to make a precise diagnosis. The clinical manifestations are non-specific and common to neoplastic effusions of other origin; the radiological aspects can be indicative only in advanced cases (e.g. in the presence of a pleural rind), and therefore in the diagnostic process, it is necessary to resort to invasive investigations. The anamnestic data of exposure to asbestos can lead to suspicion, although they are not always present. In our experience, the anamnestic data of occupational or environmental exposure to asbestos were present in only around 60% of patients.

The tools available to obtain the diagnosis are the following:

- Cytological examination of the pleural fluid
- Cyto-histological examination obtained with blind pleural biopsy
- Cyto-histological examination obtained with CT- or ultrasound-guided biopsy
- Medical Thoracoscopy
- Surgical biopsy

The cytological examination performed on the pleural fluid has a low diagnostic yield and lower than that of metastatic effusions [4]. In our experience relating to 182 patients studied from 1989 to 2015 (out of 746 Medical Thoracoscopies performed) (◘ Fig. 4.1), cytology was diagnostic only in 26.5% of cases and was positive for neoplasia but not indicative for mesothelioma in another 9.5% (◘ Fig. 4.2). Our results were similar to those of other series and in particular to those of Boutin [5].

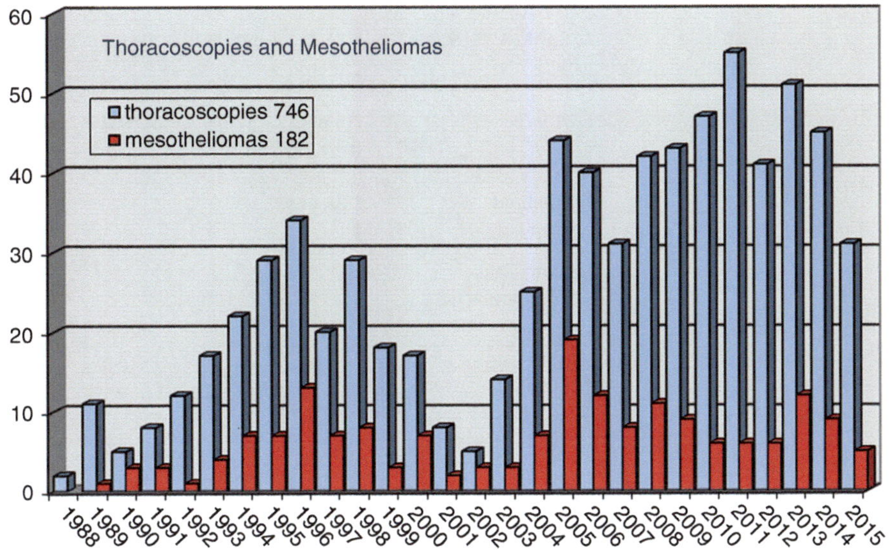

Fig. 4.1 Our experience in mesotheliomas until the end of 2015

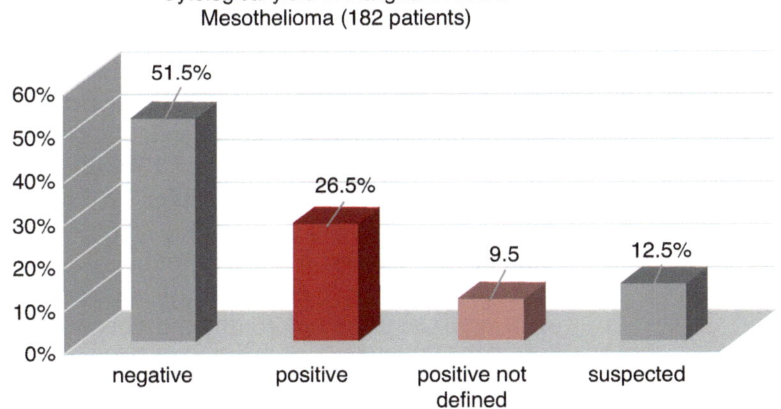

Fig. 4.2 Yield of the cytological examination in mesothelioma in our experience

In a review of another case series carried out by us in 2011 [6], most (79.1%) of the 139 malignant pleural mesotheliomas were of epithelioid histotype, a percentage slightly higher than that of ReNaM, of 55.8%; another 7.2% were sarcomatous and 10.1% biphasic (Table 4.1).

The 2010 guidelines of the ERS and ESTS [7] with 1B evidence recommend not making the diagnosis of malignant pleural mesothelioma only with cytological examination on account of the high risk of error. The use of fine needle

Table 4.1 Subdivision of the different histotypes in our experience

Histotype	Number of patients observed from 1989 to 2011	%
Epithelioid	110	79.1
• Papillary	1	0.7
Sarcomatous	10	7.2
• Desmoplastic	4	2.9
Biphasic	14	10.1
Total	139	100

biopsies is also not recommended because of its low sensitivity (<30%) and the risk of error; the 2nd Italian Consensus Conference on MPM also advises against the use of the blind biopsy [3]. With 1A evidence, on the other hand, thoracoscopy is recommended as a first choice investigation, since by means of multiple and large biopsies (no fewer than 10–15 samples), it allows us to obtain a diagnosis in over 90% of cases; the guidelines also recommend multiple samplings not only on the visibly pathological pleura but also on the apparently normal pleura. Thoracoscopy as the best investigation is also suggested by the most recent recommendations of the 3rd Italian Consensus Conference on MPM of 2016 [8]. The latest ERS/ESTS/EACTS/ESTRO guidelines [9] of 2020 suggest that the pleural biopsy with imaging guide (CT or ultrasound guide) should be used in cases where it is not possible to perform thoracoscopy, for example in the case of inaccessible pleural cavity owing to the presence of adhesions, or when thoracoscopy is not diagnostic; the diagnostic yield is about 87% compared to 47% of biopsies without imaging guide [10].

Endoscopic evaluation allows us, with high probability, to differentiate a benign from a malignant disease; it does not allow us to differentiate a primary neoplasm from a metastatic one

The appearance of the lesions highlighted by thoracoscopy is variable and not pathognomonic; in some situations, there is a macroscopic picture of chronic non-specific pleurisy; in the other situations – the most frequent – nodules of different sizes and appearance are present and it is possible to move towards a neoplastic pathology, but not to establish whether it is primitive or metastatic (■ Fig. 4.3).

Thoracoscopy, in addition to allowing for a precise diagnosis, contributes to the staging of mesothelioma especially at the initial stages (see below). At the same session, it is also possible to perform talc poudrage (see clinical case presented). The presence of sclero-hyaline pleural plaques (■ Fig. 4.4) is not a diagnostic element, but only a sign of previous exposure to asbestos. The presence of pleural plaques is associated with

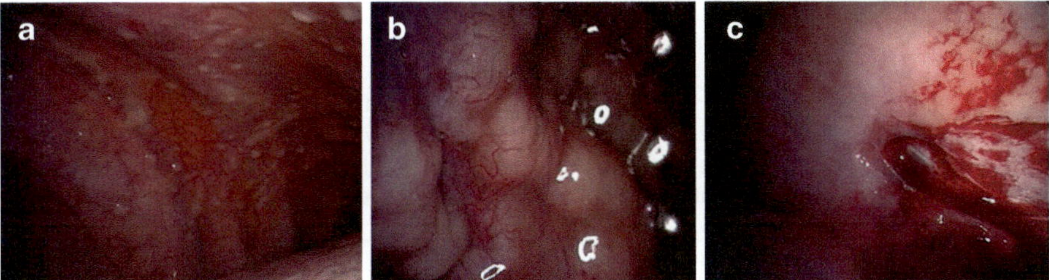

■ **Fig. 4.3** (**a**) Micronodulation, (**b**) coarse nodules, (**c**) non-specific aspect

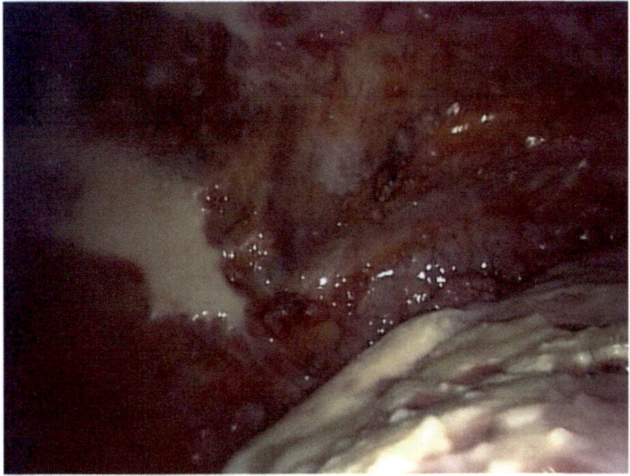

■ **Fig. 4.4** Extensive pleural plaques on the parietal pleura and diaphragmatic pleura in the left pleural cavity associated with neoplastic nodules (epithelioid mesothelioma)

a greater risk of mesothelioma and also of lung cancer and is therefore a sure sign of exposure to asbestos, but not a sign of neoplastic degeneration or precancerous disease [11].

The dosage of neoplastic markers (in particular mesothelin) in the patient's serum is still under study and of limited usefulness in the practical management of the patient; the addition of another marker (YKL-40) can improve the specificity of mesothelin [12].

The limits of thoracoscopy consist of the possible presence of false negatives (3–10%) and the difficulty or inability to explore some areas such as the mediastinal face of the visceral pleura, the pericardium and the mediastinal pleura.

Limitations of thoracoscopy:
- *3–10% of misdiagnosis*
- *areas that are difficult to explore*

The complete staging of the MPM [13] (■ Fig. 4.5) is complex and requires the use of several investigations: CT, PET, MRI, EBUS, echocardiography, mediastinoscopy and thoracotomy. The description of these investigations and their real usefulness does not fall within the scope of this manual, and therefore, please refer to the authoritative scientific literature

4

T1 T1a T1b	Ipsilateral parietal pleura No visceral pleura Visceral pleura
T2	Ipsilateral lung, diaphragm, confluent involvement of visceral pleura
T3	Endothoracic fascia, mediastinal fat, focal chest wall, non-transmural pericardium
T4	Contralateral pleura, peritoneum, rib, extensive chest wall or mediastinal invasion, myocardium, brachial plexus, spine, transmural pericardium, malignant pericardial effusion
N0	No regional lymph node metastasis
N1	Ipsilateral bronchopulmonary, hilar
N2	Subcarinal, ipsilateral mediastinal, internal mammary
N3	Contralateral mediastinal, internal mammary, hilar, ipsi/contralateral supraclavicular, scalene
M0	No extrathoracic metastasis
M1	Extrathoracic metastasis

Fig. 4.5 Summary of TNM staging in malignant pleural mesothelioma from [7]

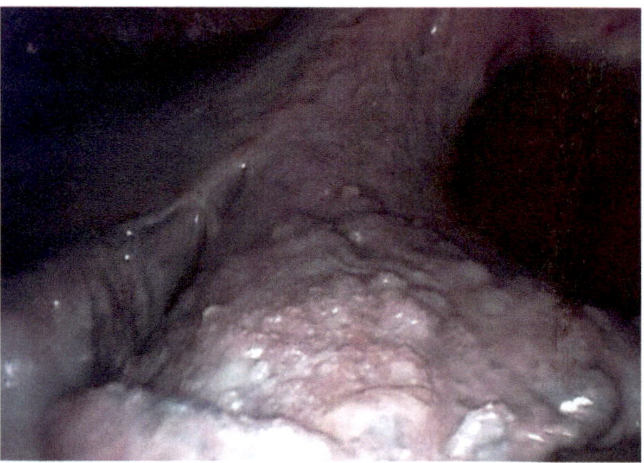

Fig. 4.6 Clear neoplastic nodulation on the surface of the left lower lobe near the fissure

for further information [8, 13, 14]. Unfortunately, in most cases, these investigations are ends unto themselves because of the poor prognosis!

It is important to reiterate that thoracoscopy plays a fundamental role in defining the initial stages; stage T1a, when the visceral pleura is free; T1b, when there are rare lesions on the visceral pleura and stage T2 (Fig. 4.6), when the involvement of the visceral pleura is extensive. In particular, the finding of a T1a or T1b stage, i.e., without localisations of the visceral pleura, could, with due reservations, lead towards a possible multimodal therapeutic approach.

In conclusion, we present a flow chart of a possible diagnostic path in a pleural effusion of suspected neoplastic nature, also applicable in the case of mesothelioma (Fig. 4.7).

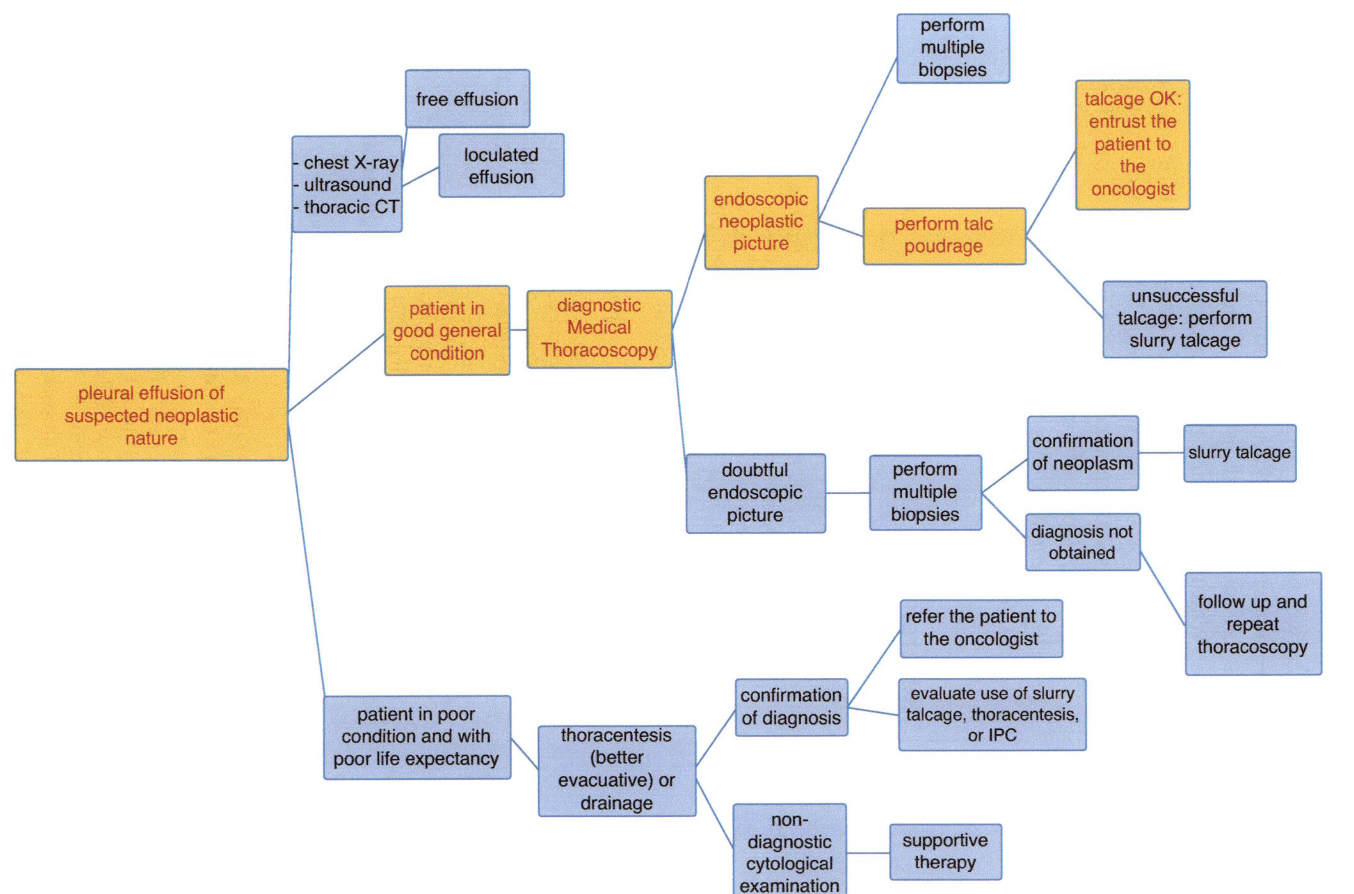

Fig. 4.7 Diagnostic-therapeutic process for a patient with pleural effusion of suspected neoplastic nature

- **Comments on the Flow Chart**

The proposed flow chart warrants the following comments:

- Why avoid thoracentesis in a patient in good general condition and able to undergo medical thoracoscopy? The answer is simple:
  - The yield of cytology is low (about 60% in metastatic effusions and about 30% in mesothelioma)
  - Waiting times for the cytological examination response are generally about 1 week: time wasted for the patient!
  - Thoracoscopy allows in over 90% of cases for a precise diagnosis and correct staging (important only for prognostic purposes in mesothelioma); above all, it is possible through talcage to solve the problem of relapses in 80% to 90% of cases!

References

1. Pinto C, Novello S, Torri V, Ardizzoni A, Betta PG, Bertazzi PA, Casalini GA, Fava C, Fubini B, Magnani C, Mirabelli D, Papotti M, Ricardi U, Rocco G, Pastorino U, Tassi G, Trodella L, Zompatori M, Scagliotti G. Second Italian consensus conference on malignant pleural mesothelioma: state of the art and recommendations. Cancer Treat Rev. 2013;39(4):328–39. https://doi.org/10.1016/j.ctrv.2012.11.004. Epub 2012 Dec 12. PMID: 23244777.
2. Il Registro Nazionale Dei Mesoteliomi. Sesto Rapporto. INAIL 2018. Collana Ricerche.
3. Montanaro F, Rosato R, Gangemi M, Roberti S, Ricceri F, Merler E, Gennaro V, Romanelli A, Chellini E, Pascucci C, Musti M, Nicita C, Barbieri PG, Marinaccio A, Magnani C, Mirabelli D. Survival of pleural malignant mesothelioma in Italy: a population-based study. Int J Cancer. 2009;124(1):201–7. https://doi.org/10.1002/ijc.23874. PMID: 18792097.
4. Tassi GF, Marchetti GP. Il versamento pleurico neoplastico primitivo (mesotelioma pleurico). In: Casalini AG, editor. Pneumologia interventistica. Milano: Springer Italia; 2007.
5. Boutin C, Rey F. Thoracoscopy in pleural malignant mesothelioma: a prospective study of 188 consecutive patients. Part 1: diagnosis. Cancer. 1993;72(2):389–93. https://doi.org/10.1002/1097-0142(19930715)72:2<389::aid-cncr2820720213>3.0.co;2-v. PMID: 8319170.
6. Casalini AG, Melioli MPA, A, Rindi G, Lasagna L, Sabbadini F, Tafuro F, Bertorelli G. Mesotelioma maligno desmoplastico: presentazione di 4 casi clinici e breve revisione della letteratura. Rassegna Patol dell'Apparato Resp. 2011;26:18–23.
7. Scherpereel A, Astoul P, Baas P, Berghmans T, Clayson H, de Vuyst P, Dienemann H, Galateau-Salle F, Hennequin C, Hillerdal G, Le Péchoux C, Mutti L, Pairon JC, Stahel R, van Houtte P, van Meerbeeck J, Waller D, Weder W, European Respiratory Society/European Society of Thoracic Surgeons Task Force. Guidelines of the European Respiratory Society and the European Society of Thoracic Surgeons

for the management of malignant pleural mesothelioma. Eur Respir J. 2010;35(3):479–95. https://doi.org/10.1183/09031936.00063109. Epub 2009 Aug 28. PMID: 19717482.

8. Novello S, Pinto C, Torri V, Porcu L, Di Maio M, Tiseo M, Ceresoli G, Magnani C, Silvestri S, Veltri A, Papotti M, Rossi G, Ricardi U, Trodella L, Rea F, Facciolo F, Granieri A, Zagonel V, Scagliotti G. The Third Italian consensus conference for malignant pleural mesothelioma: state of the art and recommendations. Crit Rev Oncol Hematol. 2016;104:9–20. https://doi.org/10.1016/j.critrevonc.2016.05.004. Epub 2016 May 13. PMID: 27286698.
9. Opitz I, Scherpereel A, Berghmans T, Psallidas I, Glatzer M, Rigau D, Astoul P, Bölükbas S, Boyd J, Coolen J, De Bondt C, De Ruysscher D, Durieux V, Faivre-Finn C, Fennell DA, Galateau-Salle F, Greillier L, Hoda MA, Klepetko W, Lacourt A, McElnay P, Maskell NA, Mutti L, Pairon JC, Van Schil P, van Meerbeeck JP, Waller D, Weder W, Putora PM, Cardillo G. ERS/ESTS/EACTS/ESTRO guidelines for the management of malignant pleural mesothelioma. Eur J Cardiothorac Surg. 2020;58(1):1–24. https://doi.org/10.1093/ejcts/ezaa158. PMID: 32448904.
10. Maskell NA, Gleeson FV, Davies RJ. Standard pleural biopsy versus CT-guided cutting-needle biopsy for diagnosis of malignant disease in pleural effusions: a randomised controlled trial. Lancet. 2003;361(9366):1326–30. https://doi.org/10.1016/s0140-6736(03)13079-6. PMID: 12711467.
11. American Thoracic Society. Diagnosis and initial management of nonmalignant diseases related to asbestos. Am J Respir Crit Care Med. 2004;170(6):691–715. https://doi.org/10.1164/rccm.200310-1436ST. PMID: 15355871.
12. Corradi M, Goldoni M, Alinovi R, Tiseo M, Ampollini L, Bonini S, Carbognani P, Casalini A, Mutti A. YKL-40 and mesothelin in the blood of patients with malignant mesothelioma, lung cancer and asbestosis. Anticancer Res. 2013;33(12):5517–24. PMID: 24324091.
13. Nowak AK. CT, RECIST, and malignant pleural mesothelioma. Lung Cancer. 2005;49(Suppl 1):S37–40. https://doi.org/10.1016/j.lungcan.2005.03.030. Epub 2005 Apr 20. PMID: 15950799.
14. Gelzinis TA. The 2019 ERS/ESTS/EACTS/ESTRO guidelines on the management of patients with malignant pleural mesothelioma. J Cardiothorac Vasc Anesth. 2021;35(2):378–88. https://doi.org/10.1053/j.jvca.2020.07.017. Epub 2020 Jul 30. PMID: 32798169.

Exudative Pleural Effusion: Secondary Neoplastic Pleural Effusion

Contents

Clinical Case of Neoplastic Pleural Effusion in Patient with Lung Cancer

Angelo G. Casalini

Contents

A. G. Casalini (ed.), *Practical Manual of Pleural Pathology*,
https://doi.org/10.1007/978-3-031-20312-1_5

We here present the case of a 56-year-old man, a heavy smoker (60 pack-years), in therapy for arterial hypertension.

For some months, he had complained of a mainly dry cough, which had been treated with inhaled bronchodilators without a spirometry being performed! In the last 15–20 days, he had presented with dyspnoea from exertion and accentuation of the cough.

He entered the emergency room, where he underwent a chest X-ray (◘ Fig. 5.1), which showed a right paratracheal pulmonary mass and a lower right homogeneous opacity with blunting of the costophrenic angle, indicative of pleural effusion, and was therefore sent to our ward.

A contrast-enhanced chest CT scan was performed (◘ Fig. 5.2).

This confirmed the presence of the right paratracheal mass and of the pleural effusion and documented the presence of pleural nodularity. The radiological picture therefore pointed without doubt towards a lung tumour of the right upper lobe with very probable pleural metastases and pleural effusion.

In a clinical situation such as this, several diagnostic options can be followed:

- It is possible to reach the lesion with a fluoroscopy-guided bronchoscopy or with R-EBUS to perform a targeted sampling: the diagnostic yield in similar cases is between 50% and 80%.
- A thoracentesis can be performed: the yield of the cytological examination in the neoplastic effusion is approximately 50–60%.

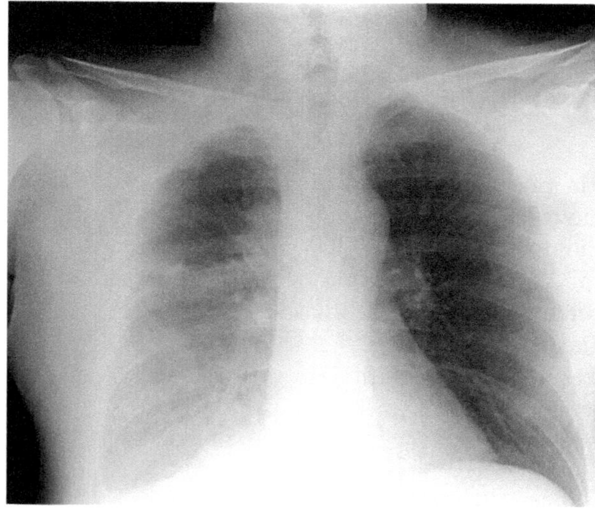

◘ **Fig. 5.1** Chest X-ray at the time of admission

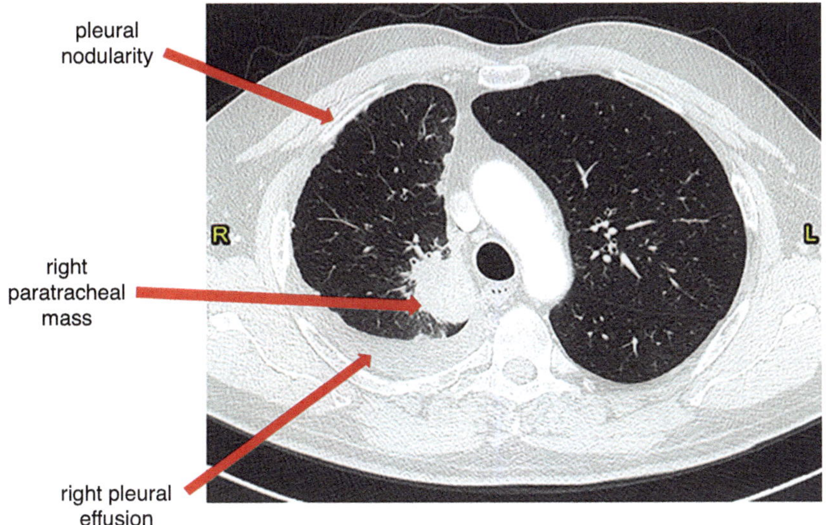

Fig. 5.2 CT of the chest

- It would be possible to perform a transthoracic fine needle aspiration of the paratracheal mass (TTNA) under CT control: diagnostic yield about 80–90%.
- CT or ultrasound-guided pleural biopsy can be performed.
- It is possible to perform a medical thoracoscopy.

In our experience in similar cases, unfortunately frequent, we have always opted for a medical thoracoscopy when the patient's clinical conditions allowed it. In this patient, it was performed on the third day of hospitalisation. Medical thoracoscopy was carried out in the endoscopy suite; the patient lay on his healthy side under local anaesthesia with 2% lidocaine and moderate sedation using midazolam, according to the technique described by Boutin [1] using a rigid 7-mm trocar (Wolf). The instrument was introduced in the left anterior axillary, after ultrasound examination.

Thoracoscopy made it possible to document with certainty the presence of pleural metastases (Fig. 5.3) (therefore stage M1a) and to take histological samples suitable for all investigations of the case (ADK with negative molecular investigations); all the pleural fluid present was evacuated, and then in the same endoscopic session, which lasted about 40 min, we performed chemical pleurodesis with talc poudrage (4 g of Steritalc-Novatech).

On the 12th day from admission, because of the lack of pleural fluid from the drain, a chest X-ray was performed (Fig. 5.4), which documented the complete resolution of

5

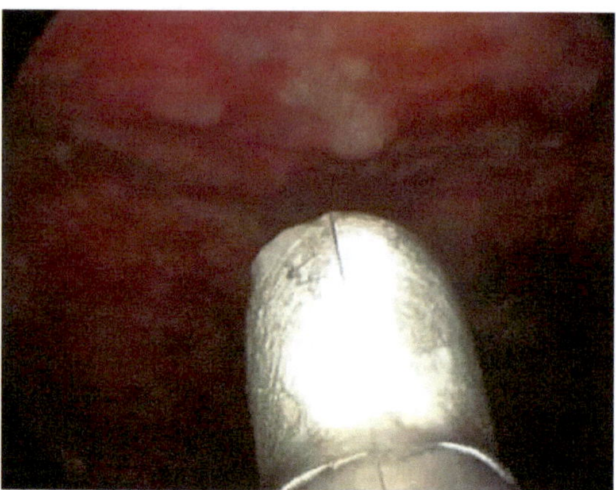

Fig. 5.3 Confirmation of the diffuse neoplastic nodularity in the right parietal pleura already highlighted on the CT scan

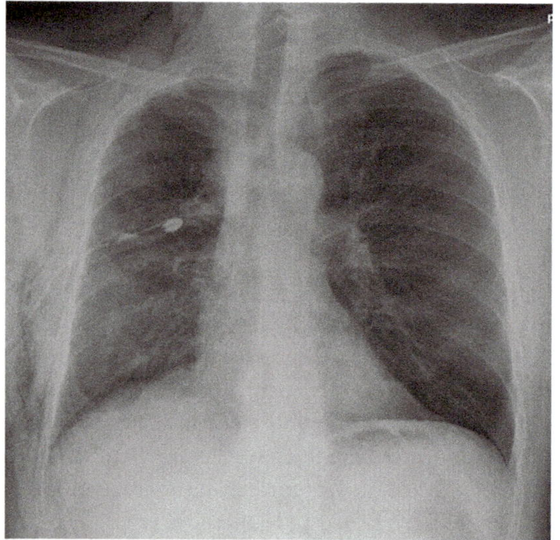

Fig. 5.4 Chest X-ray at discharge

the pleural effusion and a modest asymptomatic subcutaneous emphysema. The pleural drain was removed, and the patient was discharged and referred to the Oncologist.

The patient was followed up, and there was no resumption of the pleural effusion.

Conclusive Comments

There was the possibility to choose among different diagnostic methods; however, each of these had limitations.

In other medical environments, perhaps the patient would have followed another path, certainly longer.

The choice of the approach using medical thoracoscopy allowed us without wasting time to obtain diagnostic confirmation with suitable histological material and to solve the clinical problem of relapsing pleural effusion with talc poudrage.

Reference

1. Boutin C, Viallat JR, Aelony Y. Practical thoracoscopy. Berlin: Springer Verlag; 1991.

Secondary Neoplastic Pleural Effusion

Angelo G. Casalini

Contents

A. G. Casalini (ed.), *Practical Manual of Pleural Pathology*,
https://doi.org/10.1007/978-3-031-20312-1_6

6.1 Personal Experience

I happened to receive criticism from an oncologist because I had performed a talcage of a neoplastic effusion (it was a case of pleural metastases of a breast tumour) before entrusting her to him. He told me that the evolution of the effusion for them is an important parameter for evaluating the response to cancer therapy. I leave the reader free to comment.

6.2 Extent of the Problem

In the United States, there are over 150,000 neoplastic pleural effusions every year [1], while in Europe every year, more than 100,000 patients present a pleural effusion secondary to lung cancer [2].

Most of the exudative effusions that arrive in our wards are neoplastic

From 42% to 77% of the exudative pleural effusions that come to our attention are neoplastic [3]; these percentages vary according to the different cases, but unequivocally demonstrate clearly the reality that not only the Pulmonologist, but also the Internist and the Oncologist, have to face when dealing with a pleural effusion at the clinical onset. Most of these effusions are metastatic and in particular derive from tumours of the lung (37.5%), breast tumours (16.8%), lymphomas (11.5%), genitourinary tract tumours (9.4%) and gastrointestinal tract tumours (6.9%), as reported in the BTS guidelines [4] and deriving from 5 large series [5–9] for a total of 2040 patients (◘ Table 6.1). It is important to underline a significant datum that often comes up in our clinical experience and that is also present in this large series below: in about 10% of cases, the site of the primary tumour is not identified.

◘ Table 6.1 From the BTS guidelines [4]

Primary tumour site in 2040 patients (BTS 2010)		
	No.	**%**
Lung tumour	764	37.5
Breast tumour	343	16.8
Lymphoma	234	11.5
Genitourinary tumour	191	9.4
Gastrointestinal tumour	141	6.9
Other	148	7.8
Unknown origin	219	10.7
	2040	

Another important aspect to consider concerns the prognosis in patients with neoplastic effusion. In cases where the effusion is the first manifestation of the tumour, the average survival rate is 9.6 months [10], while it drops dramatically to 54% deaths within 1 month and 84% deaths within 6 months when the onset of the effusion is subsequent to the diagnosis of the primary tumour [11].

The prognosis for cancer effusions is poor

Regarding the most frequent neoplastic pleural effusion, that is, in lung cancer, which in the most recent revision of the staging is considered stage IV–M1a [12], Froudarakis [13] reports that its incidence varies from 7% to 23% of patients and constitutes a clearly unfavourable prognostic element. In a retrospective analysis by Porcel of 556 patients with newly diagnosed lung cancer [14], approximately 40% of patients developed pleural effusions in the course of the disease and the overall survival of patients with malignant pleural effusion was 5.49 months.

A neoplastic pleural effusion, beyond the poor prognosis *quoad vitam*, is generally very limiting and disabling for the patient (severe dyspnoea, need for repeated and frequent thoracentesis, etc.), and it is therefore imperative for the doctor to adopt all the methods that can limit or even (in most cases) solve this problem. Our goal must therefore be to do our utmost for our patients, especially when it comes to quality of life!

Pleural effusion dramatically affects the patient's quality of life!

Most patients are symptomatic and have dyspnoea of differing degrees based on the extent of the effusion and any concomitant pathologies and cough; in other patients in whom the effusion is metastatic, the symptoms of the primary tumour may already be present. The clinical situations that occur in practice are the following:

- patients with lung cancer (most frequent situation) already known and progressing, or at the clinical onset, as in the clinical case presented;
- patients with metastases of another neoplasm, usually already known, for example breast cancer in women, in which the effusion can appear even after some time, or as an onset without anamnestic data of previous malignancy elsewhere;
- patients with suspected mesothelioma.

In patients with lung cancer [15], the effusion in most cases is metastatic and is linked to the spread to the pleura of the neoplasm (stage M1a), but it can also be paraneoplastic and caused by lymphatic obstruction, post-obstructive pneumonia or atelectasis. In other situations, it may have no relationship with the neoplasm but may be caused by heart failure, infections, hypoproteinemia or pulmonary embolism; hence, there

Some pleural effusions that accompany lung cancer are not metastatic!

is the need for a correct diagnostic framework. Thoracoscopy in this case therefore plays an important role as it can demonstrate whether the effusion is neoplastic or not, it enables us to avoid an exploratory thoracotomy, and during the same procedure, it is possible to perform talc poudrage [15].

6.3 Diagnosis

The suspicion of a neoplastic effusion must always be considered in a patient with unilateral pleural effusion! A dedicated diagnostic path must therefore be followed, such as that of the flow chart presented in ◘ Fig. 6.1.

Generally, the diagnostic process involves thoracentesis as the most important manoeuvre to search for neoplastic cells.

In our experience, this approach is not always the most correct, and in many clinical situations, as in the clinical case presented, we chose, for various reasons that will be reiterated and explained later, to start with Medical Thoracoscopy.

It is important to know the limits of cytological diagnosis

The cytological examination of the pleural fluid is diagnostic in about 58% of cases [16]. Other authors [17] report a lower diagnostic sensitivity overall, of 46% of 515 patients; however, this last case series also includes 148 mesotheliomas, in which the yield of the cytological examination is lower; the same authors conclude that the repetition of the cytological examination with subsequent thoracentesis does not significantly contribute to improving the diagnostic yield. Needle pleural biopsy without imaging guidance adds little to the diagnosis (◘ Table 6.2) [16].

In a large review of the literature [18] which included 14 clinical studies with 2893 pleural biopsies performed with Abrams needle without radiological guidance, the diagnostic yield was 57% in neoplastic pleural effusions, therefore similar to that of cytology, while it was 75% in tuberculous pleural effusions. This wide difference is easily explained by the different involvement of the parietal pleura in the two different pathologies; extended to almost the entire pleural surface in TB (◘ Fig. 6.2a), or with sparing of large free areas in neoplastic pleurisy, as in this case of deciduous malignant pleural mesothelioma (◘ Fig. 6.2b) [19].

The use of the CT guide [20] enables us to reach a diagnostic sensitivity of 87% with a negative predictive value (NPV) of 80%.

The diagnosis of neoplastic effusion therefore requires confirmation of a positive cytological examination in the pleural fluid or a histological examination on a pleural biopsy. If

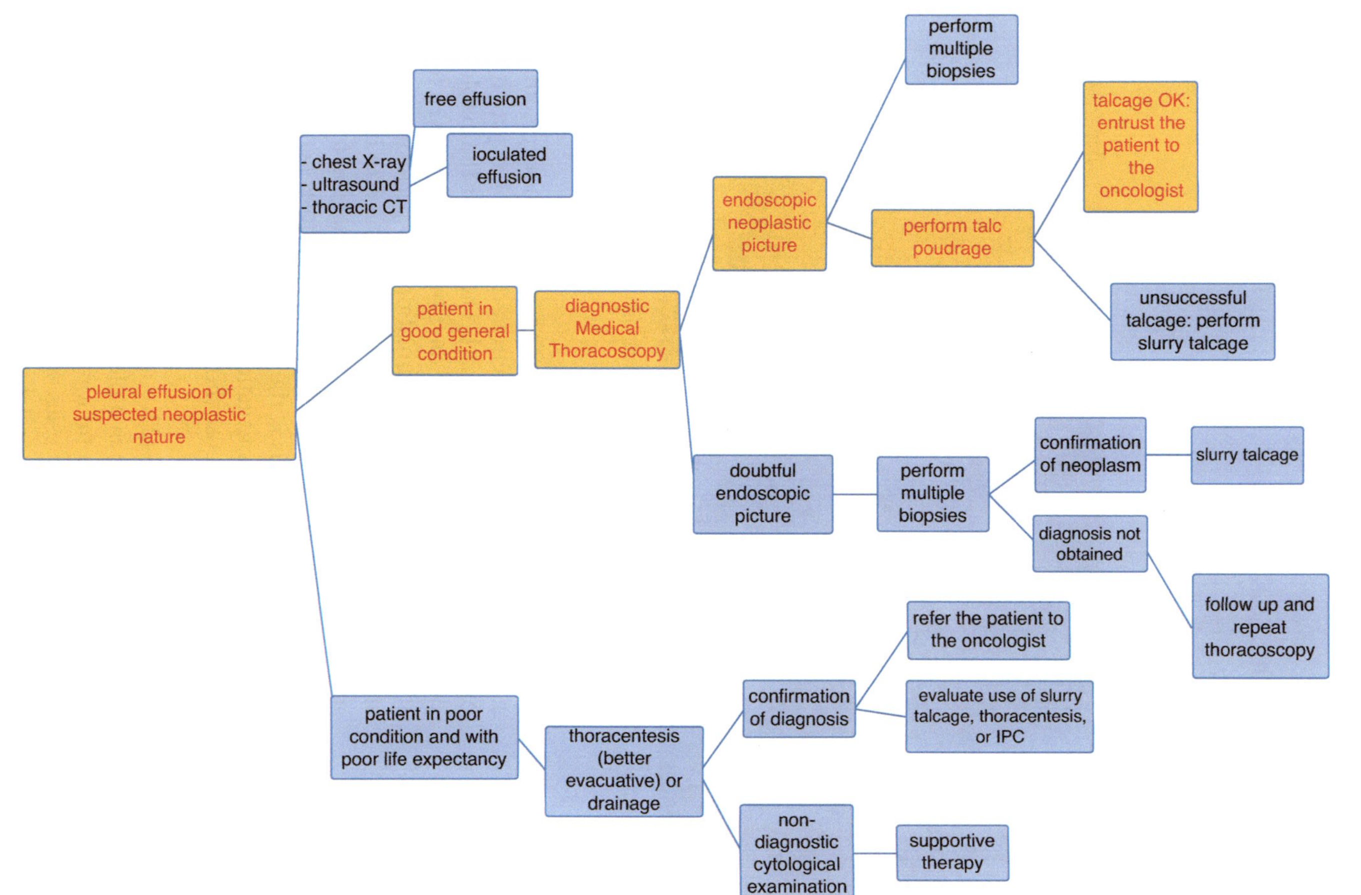

Fig. 6.1 Diagnostic-therapeutic flow chart

Table 6.2 From Prakash [16]

Investigation	No.	%
Cytology	163/281	58
Pleural needle biopsy	121/281	43
cytology + biopsy	183/281	65

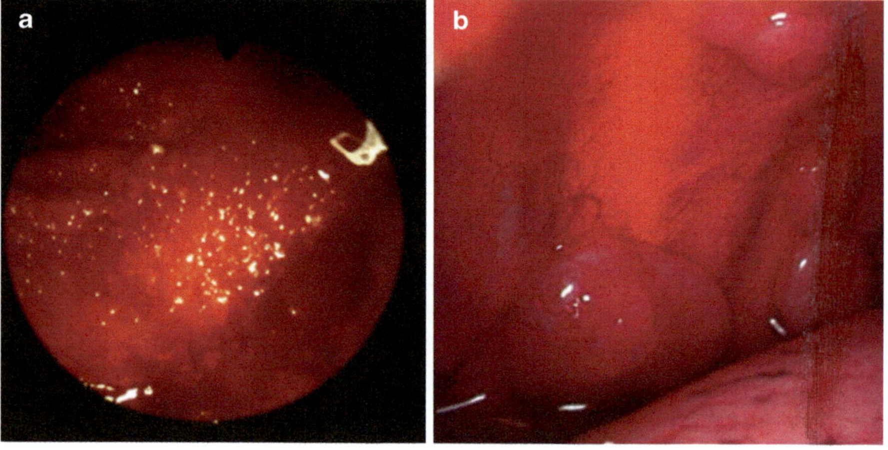

Fig. 6.2 (**a**) Endoscopic picture of tuberculous pleurisy; (**b**) deciduous malignant pleural mesothelioma

the suspicion of neoplasm is strong, some authors recommend a second thoracentesis and then, in the case of negativity, the execution of a thoracoscopy [21]. The wait for the cytological diagnosis can take from 5 to 7 days (in some cases even longer if immunohistochemical investigations are performed); in the meantime, the patient remains symptomatic and it is reasonable to question whether this behaviour is logical and whether it is correct to extend the time of the diagnosis pending a further thoracentesis! This is the main reason why, in the strong suspicion of a neoplastic aetiology of the pleural effusion, in many situations we choose thoracoscopy as the first diagnostic investigation.

Medical Thoracoscopy is the investigation of choice in diagnosing a suspected neoplastic effusion

The BTS guidelines [22] emphasise that thoracoscopy is the investigation of choice in a pleural effusion in which cytology is not conclusive and a tumour is suspected. It is also possible to perform pleural biopsies with dedicated needles (Abrams and Cope), better under CT or ultrasound control. Comparisons between pleural biopsies under imaging control (CT or echo) and thoracoscopy [23], while demonstrating a

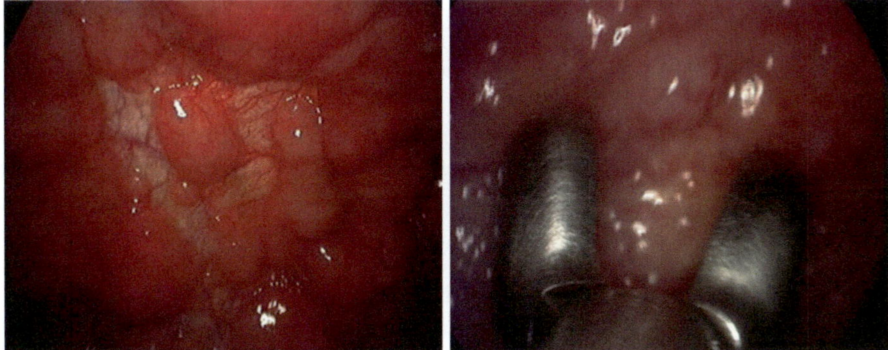

■ **Fig. 6.3** Neoplastic nodules from pulmonary ADK metastases: targeted biopsy

high diagnostic sensitivity of needle biopsies, conclude that thoracoscopy is superior, with a sensitivity of 94.1 compared to 87.5%; endoscopic vision allows for targeted biopsies (■ Fig. 6.3).

So we reiterate that in our experience we do not use needle pleural biopsies, and when there is a strong suspicion of neoplasia, we think it is useless for the patient to wait a long time for the cytological diagnosis on the pleural fluid; in many cases, as in the clinical case presented before this chapter, we choose medical thoracoscopy as the first diagnostic approach for its high diagnostic yield (greater than 95%) and for the possibility of associating pleurodesis (see clinical case); see the flow chart of ■ Fig. 6.1.

Always consider the diagnostic aspect and the therapeutic aspect as being associated!

It is therefore essential in approaching the patient not to consider only the diagnostic aspect but also the possibility of providing an indispensable treatment such as pleurodesis. The advantage of being able to perform thoracoscopic talcage, considered superior to slurry, and at the same time to obtain the precise diagnosis in patients who have a highly suspected neoplastic pleural effusion, justifies this approach. This opinion is shared by other authors [24]. If we consider that the only way to improve the quality of life of patients with neoplastic pleural effusion is the control of dyspnoea through talcage, this seems to us the most rational approach.

6.4 Therapeutic Interventions

Therapeutic interventions are aimed at improving the patient's quality of life [25] and are:

- Evacuative thoracentesis
- Chest drainage

- Pleurodesis
- IPC (indwelling pleural catheter)
- The pleuroperitoneal shunt

The choice of the most appropriate intervention depends on many factors, related not only to the patient but also to the habits and skills of the doctor who must manage the patient. What is certain is that the more competent the doctor, the more the patient will benefit.

The flow chart of ◘ Fig. 6.1 suggests which strategy could be followed in our opinion, validated by a long clinical experience. The two fundamental criteria that guide a therapeutic decision are: clinical improvement after thoracentesis, when this is performed as the first investigation, and a good life expectancy for the patient.

6.5 Thoracentesis

Thoracentesis is not always followed by clinical improvement with complete or partial remission of dyspnoea. The latter is often multifactorial and may depend on an underlying cardiopulmonary disease, pneumonia or tumour-related complications such as pulmonary embolism, bronchial obstruction or carcinomatous lymphangitis.

Thoracentesis: indispensable and safe investigation in particular with ultrasound guidance

Thoracentesis, especially if performed under ultrasound guidance, is a safe investigation with very rare complications [26]. However, thoracentesis can present some problems; repeated discomfort for the patient, particularly in effusions that re-form rapidly and require repeated visits to the hospital for frequent thoracentesis; possible complications related to the manoeuvre: pneumothorax, cardiovascular collapse, *ex vacuo* pulmonary oedema, infection of the cavity, or possible malignant seeding in the case of mesothelioma. It is important to remember that these pleural fluids are rich in proteins (up to 40–50 g/L) and that often 2–3 L of fluid per week are formed in these patients; this continuous and strong loss of proteins contributes to the evolution of the patient's cachectic state.

6.6 Pleurodesis

When possible, perform pleurodesis without unnecessary waiting

Certainly, when feasible, pleurodesis is the method of choice and is the one recommended by the guidelines [4, 27] as it can be a 'definitive' intervention that solves the problem of relapses. The goal is to obtain a symphysis between the two pleural sheets (parietal and visceral) with the aim of limiting or completely avoiding the production of fluid. The methods for obtaining a symphysis can be mechanical or physical, directed on the parietal pleura by mechanical abrasion, laser or argon beam coagulation or by administering various substances: talc (thoracoscopically or through a drainage tube), bleomycin or tetracyclines. Generally, the most used substance is talc through the thoracoscopic route (talc poudrage) or through the drainage tube (talc slurry). The advantage of thoracoscopic talc poudrage is that it can be performed directly during the thoracoscopy, through which a direct exploration of the pleural cavity can be performed, eliminating any adhesions that would prevent a complete diffusion of the talc, pulverising the talc therefore in a targeted way and on the dry pleura [28].

As regards the mechanism by which pleurodesis occurs, please refer to the specific literature [29]. It should be remembered that some parameters, including the pH of the pleural fluid, can be predictive of the success of talcage; Rodriguez Panadero [30] obtained a valid pleurodesis in 79% of patients with pH > 7.30, while talcage failed when the pH was <7.15; this is because there is a direct correlation between the extension of the neoplasm and the low pH value. Thoracoscopic talcage is a safe method; 557 patients were included in a major multicentre study in whom talc poudrage was performed thoracoscopically with 4 g of French talc (Novatech Steritalc) [31], and none of them developed ARDS after talcage.

Question: first the talcage or first the oncological therapies?

A frequent and important question is whether talcage should precede or follow oncological therapies. There are no guidelines that recommend prioritising anticancer therapies before palliative treatments [27]; the only exception in our experience is lymphoma. In any case, there are no randomised/controlled studies that compare the results obtained using talcage before or after anticancer therapies or that demonstrate that talcage performed in advance can adversely affect the outcome of oncological treatments. Our experience has always been aimed at promptly intervening with talcage to improve the patient's symptoms and allow him to face the oncological therapies, avoiding unnecessary waiting!

6.7 Prognostic Factors

It is important to identify patients with a negative prognosis to avoid invasive and not really clinically useful interventions. The survival of patients with neoplastic pleural effusions varies from case to case and it may be useful to employ an easy-to-use tool to assess patient prognosis. The LENT score [32] is the first validated risk stratification system to predict the survival of patients with cancer. It is calculated on the basis of 4 simple parameters: (L) LDH in pleural fluid, (E) patient performance score (Eastern Cooperative Oncology Group (ECOG) performance score), (N) neutrophil/lymphocyte ratio in blood and (T) the type of tumour. This score, which can be easily calculated, can be a valid clinical aid in choosing the therapeutic strategy to follow and provides more precise indications than using the Performance Score alone. In high-risk patients with a high LENT Score [5–7], survival at 6 months varies from 3% to 17%, and therefore, a therapeutic approach, as little invasive as possible, such as repeated thoracentesis or the placement of an intrapleural catheter, may be advisable.

The indications as to the best therapeutic strategy to follow derive from authoritative guidelines that have been published on the subject and from the Cochrane studies; a summary of the most relevant recommendations is provided here below.

6.8 Guidelines

- The BTS guidelines [3] recommend talc as the most effective agent for pleurodesis; in the case of failure, a tunnelled catheter can be placed.
- For ERS/EACTS [27], talc is the most effective and most uncomplicated pleurodetic agent. Thoracoscopic talcage may be more effective than slurry. Surgical procedures of pleurodesis are no more effective than talcage: on the contrary, in mesothelioma in particular, they are burdened by more complications and by a more prolonged hospitalisation. The use of large-bore drains (24 F) is associated with greater success.
- For the ATS [33], in the neoplastic pleural effusion and with re-expandable lung, thoracoscopic or slurry talcage or an IPC must be performed.

6.9 Cochrane

- Cochrane 2004 [34]: talc is the most effective substance.
- Cochrane 2020 [35]: for those interested, please note that it is a 310-page document! The first review was published in 2016, and this is the latest updated review. In a nutshell, the conclusions are the following:
  - Talcage, poudrage or slurry, is the best method to carry out a pleurodesis, better than doxycycline or bleomycin.

- The thoracoscopic talcage procedure that allows for complete removal of pleural fluid and diffuse talc poudrage is probably the best technique.
- IPC is a valid alternative, limiting the use of repeated interventions (thoracentesis) and improving the patient's dyspnoea.
- In any case, the choice of the best treatment depends on local availability, on the skills of the operators, and also on the patient's choices

6.10 IPC

The use of a tunnelled pleural catheter is also gaining ground in Italy. We have no experience of this method and we can only report what is present in the literature. There is an indication for its use in particular situations: for example, in the case of talcage failure and in the case of trapped lung. In a recent review [36] which collected data from 19 clinical studies involving 1370 patients, it was concluded that the catheter achieved clinical improvement in approximately 95% of patients without significant complications. Other works confirm this result [37].

6.11 Thoracic Drainage

In the chapter dedicated to drainage, the topic on the different types of drain that can be used and their relative advantages and disadvantages will be explored. In particular, the placement of small-bore drains (such as pigtails) allows for good management, even at home, of neoplastic pleural effusions.

According to literature data and our experience, we can conclude that the thoracoscopic approach, without unnecessary loss of time harmful to the patient, is the most rational way to manage patients with neoplastic pleural effusions. It allows for a precise diagnosis in almost 95% of patients, and thoracoscopic talcage is the method recognised as the best in the literature and international guidelines.

In any case, we agree with the conclusions of the ATS guidelines: use the talcage method you prefer, but do it without wasting time!!!

References

1. Light RW. Pleural diseases. 4th ed. Philadelphia: Lippincott Williams & Wilkins; 2001.

2. Ferlay J, Autier P, Boniol M, Heanue M, Colombet M, Boyle P. Estimates of the cancer incidence and mortality in Europe in 2006. Ann Oncol. 2007;18(3):581–92. https://doi.org/10.1093/annonc/mdl498. Epub 2007 Feb 7. PMID: 17287242.
3. Sahn SA. State of the art. The pleura. Am Rev Respir Dis. 1988;138(1):184–234. https://doi.org/10.1164/ajrccm/138.1.184. PMID: 3059866.
4. Roberts ME, Neville E, Berrisford RG, Antunes G, Ali NJ, BTS Pleural Disease Guideline Group. Management of a malignant pleural effusion: British Thoracic Society Pleural Disease Guideline 2010. Thorax. 2010;65(Suppl 2):32–40. https://doi.org/10.1136/thx.2010.136994. PMID: 20696691.
5. Salyer WR, Eggleston JC, Erozan YS. Efficacy of pleural needle biopsy and pleural fluid cytopathology in the diagnosis of malignant neoplasm involving the pleura. Chest. 1975;67(5):536–9. https://doi.org/10.1378/chest.67.5536. PMID: 1126189.
6. Chernow B, Sahn SA. Carcinomatous involvement of the pleura: an analysis of 96 patients. Am J Med. 1977;63(5):695–702. https://doi.org/10.1016/0002-9343(77)90154-1. PMID: 930945.
7. Johnston WW. The malignant pleural effusion. A review of cytopathologic diagnoses of 584 specimens from 472 consecutive patients. Cancer. 1985;56(4):905–9. https://doi.org/10.1002/1097-0142(19850815)56:4<905::aid-cncr2820560435>3.0.co;2-u. PMID: 4016683.
8. Sears D, Hajdu SI. The cytologic diagnosis of malignant neoplasms in pleural and peritoneal effusions. Acta Cytol. 1987;31(2):85–97. PMID: 3469856.
9. Hsu C. Cytologic detection of malignancy in pleural effusion: a review of 5,255 samples from 3,811 patients. Diagn Cytopathol. 1987;3(1):8–12. https://doi.org/10.1002/dc.2840030103. PMID: 3568976.
10. Monte SA, Ehya H, Lang WR. Positive effusion cytology as the initial presentation of malignancy. Acta Cytol. 1987;31(4):448–52. PMID: 3604540.
11. van de Molengraft FJ, Vooijs GP. Survival of patients with malignancy-associated effusions. Acta Cytol. 1989;33(6):911–6. PMID: 2588923.
12. Detterbeck FC, Boffa DJ, Kim AW, Tanoue LT. The eighth edition lung cancer stage classification. Chest. 2017;151(1):193–203. https://doi.org/10.1016/j.chest.2016.10.010. Epub 2016 Oct 22. PMID: 27780786.
13. Froudarakis ME. Pleural effusion in lung cancer: more questions than answers. Respiration. 2012;83(5):367–76. https://doi.org/10.1159/000338169. Epub 2012 May 7. PMID: 22584211.
14. Porcel JM, Gasol A, Bielsa S, Civit C, Light RW, Salud A. Clinical features and survival of lung cancer patients with pleural effusions. Respirology. 2015;20(4):654–9. https://doi.org/10.1111/resp.12496. Epub 2015 Feb 23. PMID: 25706291.
15. American Thoracic Society. Management of malignant pleural effusions. Am J Respir Crit Care Med. 2000;162(5):1987–2001. https://doi.org/10.1164/ajrccm.162.5.ats8-00. PMID: 11069845.
16. Prakash UB, Reiman HM. Comparison of needle biopsy with cytologic analysis for the evaluation of pleural effusion: analysis of 414 cases. Mayo Clin Proc. 1985;60(3):158–64. https://doi.org/10.1016/s0025-6196(12)60212-2. PMID: 3974296.
17. Arnold DT, De Fonseka D, Perry S, Morley A, Harvey JE, Medford A, Brett M, Maskell NA. Investigating unilateral pleural effusions: the role of cytology. Eur Respir J. 2018;52(5):1801254. https://doi.org/10.1183/13993003.01254-2018. PMID: 30262573.

18. Tomlinson JR. Invasive procedures in the diagnosis of pleural disease. Semin Respir Med. 1987;9:30–6. https://doi.org/10.1055/s-2007-1012685.
19. Ferrari L, Vignali S, Mori PA, Melioli A, Gnetti L, Silini EM, Casalini AG. Un caso clinico di mesotelioma pleurico maligno ad aspetto deciduoide. Malignant deciduoid pleural mesothelioma: a case report. Rassegna Patol dell'Apparato Resp. 2014;29:52–4.
20. Maskell NA, Gleeson FV, Davies RJ. Standard pleural biopsy versus CT-guided cutting-needle biopsy for diagnosis of malignant disease in pleural effusions: a randomised controlled trial. Lancet. 2003;361(9366):1326–30. https://doi.org/10.1016/s0140-6736(03)13079-6. PMID: 12711467.
21. Noceti P, Nosenzo M. Versamento pleurico maligno secondario. In: Casalini AG, editor. Pneumologia interventistica. Milano: Springer Italia; 2007.
22. Hooper C, Lee YC, Maskell N, BTS Pleural Guideline Group. Investigation of a unilateral pleural effusion in adults: British Thoracic Society Pleural Disease Guideline 2010. Thorax. 2010;65(Suppl 2):4–17. https://doi.org/10.1136/thx.2010.136978. PMID: 20696692.
23. Metintas M, Ak G, Dundar E, Yildirim H, Ozkan R, Kurt E, Erginel S, Alatas F, Metintas S. Medical thoracoscopy vs CT scan-guided Abrams pleural needle biopsy for diagnosis of patients with pleural effusions: a randomized, controlled trial. Chest. 2010;137(6):1362–8. https://doi.org/10.1378/chest.09-0884. Epub 2010 Feb 12. PMID: 20154079.
24. Tschopp JM, Schnyder JM, Astoul P, Noppen M, Froudarakis M, Bolliger CT, Gasparini S, Tassi GF, Rodriguez-Panadero F, Loddenkemper R, Aelony Y, Janssen JP. Pleurodesis by talc poudrage under simple medical thoracoscopy: an international opinion. Thorax. 2009;64(3):273–4; author reply 274. PMID: 19252034.
25. Thomas R, Francis R, Davies HE, Lee YC. Interventional therapies for malignant pleural effusions: the present and the future. Respirology. 2014;19(6):809–22. https://doi.org/10.1111/resp.12328. Epub 2014 Jun 19. PMID: 24947955.
26. Jones PW, Moyers JP, Rogers JT, Rodriguez RM, Lee YC, Light RW. Ultrasound-guided thoracentesis: is it a safer method? Chest. 2003;123(2):418–23. https://doi.org/10.1378/chest.123.2.418. PMID: 12576360.
27. Bibby AC, Dorn P, Psallidas I, Porcel JM, Janssen J, Froudarakis M, Subotic D, Astoul P, Licht P, Schmid R, Scherpereel A, Rahman NM, Cardillo G, Maskell NA. ERS/EACTS statement on the management of malignant pleural effusions. Eur Respir J. 2018;52(1):1800349. https://doi.org/10.1183/13993003.00349-2018. PMID: 30054348.
28. Tassi GF, Marchetti GP, Bosio G. Pleurodesi toracoscopica. In: Pneumologia interventistica. Milano: Springer Italia; 2007.
29. Mierzejewski M, Korczynski P, Krenke R, Janssen JP. Chemical pleurodesis - a review of mechanisms involved in pleural space obliteration. Respir Res. 2019;20(1):247. https://doi.org/10.1186/s12931-019-1204-x. PMID: 31699094; PMCID: PMC6836467.
30. Rodríguez-Panadero F, López MJ. Low glucose and pH levels in malignant pleural effusions. Diagnostic significance and prognostic value in respect to pleurodesis. Am Rev Respir Dis. 1989;139(3):663–7. https://doi.org/10.1164/ajrccm/139.3.663. PMID: 2923367.
31. Janssen JP, Collier G, Astoul P, Tassi GF, Noppen M, Rodriguez-Panadero F, Loddenkemper R, Herth FJ, Gasparini S, Marquette CH, Becke B, Froudarakis ME, Driesen P, Bolliger CT, Tschopp JM. Safety of pleurodesis with talc poudrage in malignant pleural effusion: a pro-

spective cohort study. Lancet. 2007;369(9572):1535–9. https://doi.org/10.1016/S0140-6736(07)60708-9. PMID: 17482984.

32. Clive AO, Kahan BC, Hooper CE, Bhatnagar R, Morley AJ, Zahan-Evans N, Bintcliffe OJ, Boshuizen RC, Fysh ET, Tobin CL, Medford AR, Harvey JE, van den Heuvel MM, Lee YC, Maskell NA. Predicting survival in malignant pleural effusion: development and validation of the LENT prognostic score. Thorax. 2014;69(12):1098–104. https://doi.org/10.1136/thoraxjnl-2014-205285. Epub 2014 Aug 6. PMID: 25100651; PMCID: PMC4251306.
33. Feller-Kopman DJ, Reddy CB, DeCamp MM, Diekemper RL, Gould MK, Henry T, Iyer NP, Lee YCG, Lewis SZ, Maskell NA, Rahman NM, Sterman DH, Wahidi MM, Balekian AA. Management of malignant pleural effusions. An official ATS/STS/STR clinical practice guideline. Am J Respir Crit Care Med. 2018;198(7):839–49. https://doi.org/10.1164/rccm.201807-1415ST. PMID: 30272503.
34. Shaw P, Agarwal R. Pleurodesis for malignant pleural effusions. Cochrane Database Syst Rev. 2004;1:CD002916. https://doi.org/10.1002/14651858.CD002916.pub2. Update in: Cochrane Database Syst Rev. 2013;11:CD002916. PMID: 14973997.
35. Dipper A, Jones HE, Bhatnagar R, Preston NJ, Maskell N, Clive AO. Interventions for the management of malignant pleural effusions: a network meta-analysis. Cochrane Database Syst Rev. 2020;4(4):CD010529. https://doi.org/10.1002/14651858.CD010529.pub3. PMID: 32315458; PMCID: PMC7173736.
36. Van Meter ME, McKee KY, Kohlwes RJ. Efficacy and safety of tunneled pleural catheters in adults with malignant pleural effusions: a systematic review. J Gen Intern Med. 2011;26(1):70–6. https://doi.org/10.1007/s11606-010-1472-0. Epub 2010 Aug 10. PMID: 20697963; PMCID: PMC3024099.
37. Zahid I, Routledge T, Billè A, Scarci M. What is the best treatment for malignant pleural effusions? Interact Cardiovasc Thorac Surg. 2011;12(5):818–23. https://doi.org/10.1510/icvts.2010.254789. Epub 2011 Feb 16. PMID: 21325469.

Exudative Pleural Effusion: Infectious and Tuberculous Pleural Effusion

Contents

Introduction to Infectious and Tuberculous Pleural Effusion

Angelo G. Casalini

Contents

A. G. Casalini (ed.), *Practical Manual of Pleural Pathology*,
https://doi.org/10.1007/978-3-031-20312-1_7

In many texts and scientific works, infectious and tuberculous pleural effusions are treated separately because of their very different aetiologies and clinical-therapeutic courses. Also in this manual, they will be treated in two separate chapters, but a common introduction is required owing to the strong similarities they may present at the beginning on a clinical level. The diagnostic path that we present at the beginning is common, but subsequently divides into two different paths.

We begin this important topic by reporting our experience relating to a significant part of our clinical case history. In the period from 1 January 2001 to 31 December 2015, at our Department of Pulmonology, we treated 254 patients with infectious pleural effusion (◘ Table 7.1). Two patients with aspergillus pleural effusion were excluded from this series: They were immunosuppressed haematological neoplastic patients.

Two facts need to be highlighted.

34.2% of parapneumonic effusions were complicated or empyema

The first is that as many as 87/254 (34.2%) parapneumonic effusions were complicated or empyema effusions; therefore, thoracentesis and measurement of the pleural fluid pH are fundamental in the evaluation.

20.5% of patients had tuberculous effusions!

Another relevant fact from our experience that should be emphasised is the fact that 52/254 patients (20.5%) were affected by tuberculous pleurisy; in these patients, only a dedicated diagnostic approach, which also included medical thoracoscopy, enabled a correct diagnosis. These two topics will be taken up and expanded in their respective chapters.

We believe that this premise is important, as unfortunately sometimes thoracentesis is performed too late in parapneumonic effusions. Another important fact is the higher incidence of tuberculous effusions found by us in Parma compared with that of other experiences, both pneumological and not; therefore, tuberculous effusions are there and must be sought!

◘ **Table 7.1** Our experience of 254 infectious pleural effusions

254 patients with infectious pleural effusion from 1 January 2001 to 31 December 2015		
	No.	**%**
Simple parapneumonic effusion	115	45.3
Complicated parapneumonic effusion and empyema	87	34.2
Tuberculous pleural effusion	52	20.5
	254	

Tuberculous pleural effusions can resolve spontaneously

It was well known even before the discovery of anti-tuberculous drugs that many tuberculous effusions resolved spontaneously, and this made the fortune of our "phthisiologist" predecessors, who practically treated tuberculous pleurisy without having dedicated drugs; sometimes their treatment worked and sometimes it didn't! Also Sahn [1] reports that a tuberculous effusion can resolve spontaneously without specific therapy in 2 to 4 months! The problem is that in many patients tuberculosis relapses can actually occur with other clinical manifestations after some time [2]. If the tuberculous effusions are not sought with "obstinacy" and following a correct path, they can be missed and then open the way to possible long-term consequences, as also reported by us [3].

Too much importance is given to the search for M. tuberculosis in the pleural fluid

In the dedicated chapter, it will be demonstrated that the correct diagnosis of tuberculous effusion cannot be limited to what is "usually" performed in our hospitals; the search for *M. tuberculosis* on the pleural fluid, with smear microscopy for AFB, TB-NAAT and culture, is usually requested, but if it is negative, tuberculous pleurisy is unfortunately ruled out!

The correct clinical assessment of pleural effusion allows us in most cases to hypothesise whether it is an "infectious" pleural effusion or of another aetiology, in most cases neoplastic. When the clinical onset is characterised by fever, stinging chest pain and cough and the laboratory data are compatible, it is possible to move towards an infectious aetiology; however, it should be considered that in elderly and/or debilitated patients, the symptoms can be more veiled and subtle.

7.1 Types of Infectious Effusions, Aetiology and Related Problems

The different types of pleural effusions of infectious aetiology are summarised in ◘ Table 7.2, and many of these are actually rare.

The problems that usually occur in the management of the infectious pathology of the pleura are the following:

- The isolation of pathogens is not easy and with traditional laboratory investigations the yield in many experiences is less than 40%; it is possible to use more complex methods (molecular investigations by means of gene amplification tests) which, however, are not available in all hospitals.

Are viral pleural effusions in adults a real problem and are they not recognised or are they a "wastebasket" diagnosis?

- Unfortunately, microbiological tests are not always requested or are only partially requested; in the case of negative samples, the aetiology tends to be attributed to viruses! However, viral pleurisy in adults is truly exceptional, and therefore, the diagnosis of viral pleurisy is often

Table 7.2 Infectious effusions

Parapneumonic effusions
• simple parapneumonic effusion
• complicated parapneumonic effusion and empyema
Tuberculous pleural effusion
• simple pleuritis
• empyema
Atypical pleuritis (often opportunistic infections in immunosuppressed patients)
• fungi: candida, aspergillus, cryptococcus, coccidioides, histoplasma, blastomyces, sporothrix
• unusual bacteria: actinomyces, nocardia, chlamidia, rickettsia
• parasites: amoebiasis, echinococcosis, paragonimiasis, trichomoniasis
• virus (we don't know the real epidemiology!): adenovirus, hantavirus, cytomegalovirus, herpes virus, hepatitis, mononucleosis, dengue, influenza, parainfluenza, coxsackie viruses

a "wastebasket" diagnosis, which should always be treated with suspicion until a certain and confirmed diagnosis is made. Case reports of pleural effusion associated with SARS-CoV2 infection have recently been reported. A recent work shows extensive experience involving 153 patients with COVID-19 and pleural effusion [4]. Patients with pleural effusions had a higher incidence of severe diseases and higher mortality with longer hospital stay than patients without pleural effusion; therefore, the presence of effusion was a negative prognostic factor. This study, however, has major limitations as it reports that because of the modest amount of effusion, thoracentesis was not performed! Therefore, the study does not go into detail as to the real cause of the effusion, and it is not possible to know if it was related to infection by the virus or to other concomitant causes (e.g. heart failure).

When choosing antibiotic therapy, do not use the Pneumonia Guidelines, but those of the BTS dedicated to infectious effusion

- The aetiological agents of parapneumonic effusions and empyema are believed to be the same as for pneumonia, although the scientific literature is rich in important works that often suggest different aetiologies. This must always be considered to start a correct antibiotic therapy; therefore in

the choice of antibiotic therapy, it is not appropriate to follow the pneumonia guidelines, but those dedicated to infectious effusion as indicated by the BTS [5].
- A common mistake is the failure to distinguish simple parapneumonic effusions from complicated ones and empyema, for which different diagnostic-therapeutic approaches must be followed, as will be explained in the dedicated chapter; unfortunately, thoracentesis is often performed too late… and we will not tire of saying this in this manual!
- The real incidence of tuberculous pleural effusion is underestimated, mainly because too much importance is given to the search for *M. tuberculosis* in the pleural fluid and in particular to its negativity; a dedicated diagnostic approach will be presented in the chapter on tuberculous pleural effusion.

The following flow chart (◘ Fig. 7.1) constitutes a reasoned approach to pleural effusion of suspected infectious aetiology.

Differential cell count can play an important role

An important diagnostic step that unfortunately is neglected in many hospitals is that of the differential cell count in the pleural fluid, which in effusions of infectious origin plays a decisive role in distinguishing the effusions of tuberculous origin from the others. An important work of 1993 [6] on the recruitment of inflammatory cells in the pleural cavity in different pathological situations had emphasised the importance of this parameter in the diagnostic setting of pleural effusion and in particular of the infectious type. Numerous previous works [7] had already underlined this aspect. In particular, the differential cell count makes it possible to distinguish infectious effusions with polymorphonuclear cells (parapneumonic effusions and empyema) from those with lymphocytes (most likely tuberculous). The tuberculous pleural effusion is a lymphocytic-type exudate in 90% of cases. Polymorphonuclear cells may be predominant in the first 2 weeks from the onset of symptoms but with a subsequent change towards lymphocyte effusion [8].

Valdes reports that in 95.2% of tuberculous pleural effusions, the percentage of lymphocytes was greater than 50%, while 95% of the infectious effusions had more than 50% of neutrophils [9]. This important aspect will be analysed further in the respective chapters.

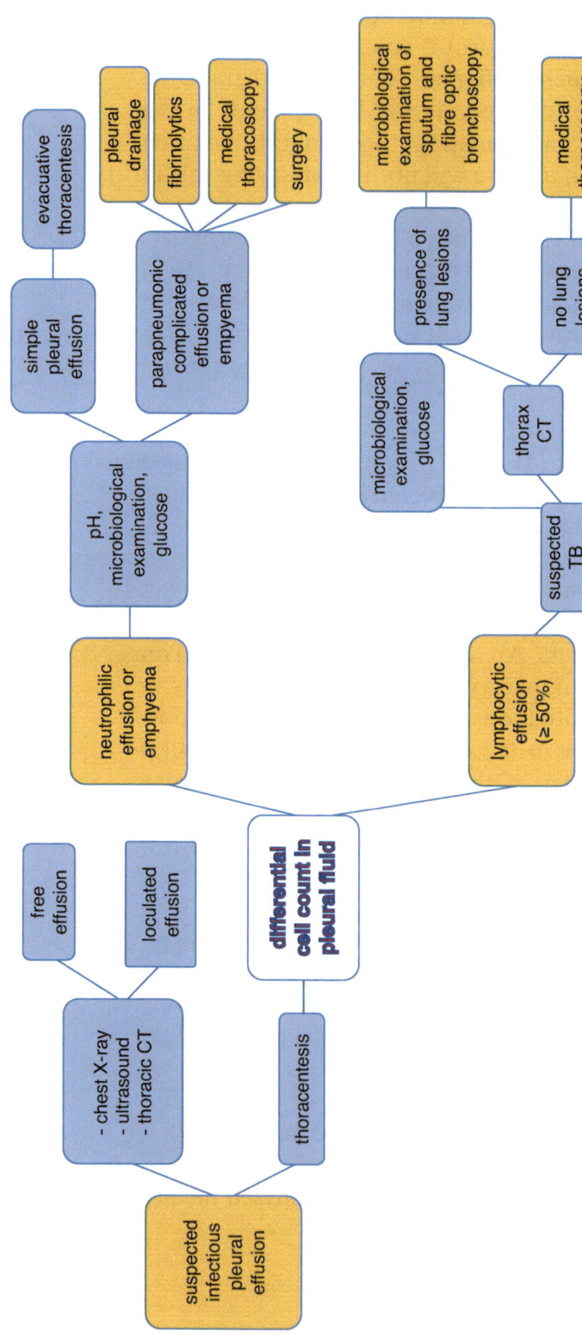

◘ Fig. 7.1 Diagnostic approach to pleural effusion of suspected infectious origin

References

1. Cohen M, Sahn SA. Resolution of pleural effusions. Chest. 2001;119(5):1547–62. https://doi.org/10.1378/chest.119.5.1547. PMID: 11348966.
2. Roper WH, Waring JJ. Primary serofibrinous pleural effusion in military personnel. Am Rev Tuberc. 1955;71(5):616–34. https://doi.org/10.1164/artpd.1955.71.5.616. PMID: 14361976.
3. Casalini AG, Cusmano F, Sverzellati N, Mori PA, Majori M. An undiagnosed pleural effusion with surprising consequences. Respir Med Case Rep. 2017;22:53–6. https://doi.org/10.1016/j.rmcr.2017.05.007. PMID: 28702335; PMCID: PMC5487223.
4. Zhan N, Guo Y, Tian S, Huang B, Tian X, Zou J, Xiong Q, Tang D, Zhang L, Dong W. Clinical characteristics of COVID-19 complicated with pleural effusion. BMC Infect Dis. 2021;21(1):176. https://doi.org/10.1186/s12879-021-05856-8. PMID: 33588779; PMCID: PMC7883764.
5. Davies HE, Davies RJ, Davies CW, BTS Pleural Disease Guideline Group. Management of pleural infection in adults: British Thoracic Society Pleural Disease Guideline 2010. Thorax. 2010;65(Suppl 2):41–53. https://doi.org/10.1136/thx.2010.137000. PMID: 20696693.
6. Antony VB, Godbey SW, Kunkel SL, Hott JW, Hartman DL, Burdick MD, Strieter RM. Recruitment of inflammatory cells to the pleural space. Chemotactic cytokines, IL-8, and monocyte chemotactic peptide-1 in human pleural fluids. J Immunol. 1993;151(12):7216–23. PMID: 8258721.
7. Spriggs AI, Boddington MM. The cytology of effusions. New York: Grune & Stratton; 1968. p. 12–40.
8. Jeon D. Tuberculous pleurisy: an update. Tuberc Respir Dis. 2014;76(4):153–9. https://doi.org/10.4046/trd.2014.76.4.153. Epub 2014 Apr 25. PMID: 24851127; PMCID: PMC4021261.
9. Valdés L, San José ME, Pose A, Gude F, González-Barcala FJ, Alvarez-Dobaño JM, Sahn SA. Diagnosing tuberculous pleural effusion using clinical data and pleural fluid analysis A study of patients less than 40 years-old in an area with a high incidence of tuberculosis. Respir Med. 2010;104(8):1211–7. https://doi.org/10.1016/j.rmed.2010.02.025. Epub 2010 Mar 26. PMID: 20347287.

First Clinical Case of Infectious Pleural Effusion

Free, Non-Loculated Effusion—Minimally Invasive Approach

Angelo G. Casalini

Contents

A. G. Casalini (ed.), *Practical Manual of Pleural Pathology*,
https://doi.org/10.1007/978-3-031-20312-1_8

We here report the case of a 34-year-old unmarried woman; a non-smoker and an office worker, she was HIV negative. Her medical history was negative. She went to the emergency department because she had been suffering from high fever and cough for 4 days, and in the last 2 days, pain had appeared in the left side of her chest, accentuated with coughing. At home, she was taking only paracetamol.

At the Emergency department, a chest X-ray (◘ Fig. 8.1) was performed, which showed a left parenchymal opacity associated with pleural effusion. The patient was sent to our ward. Physical examination of the chest revealed left posterior basal dullness with absent fremitus in the lower half of the left thorax and decreased breath sounds.

Blood tests documented marked neutrophilic leukocytosis (WBC: 16,500; neutrophils: 70%), increased ESR: 80. As is routine in these cases, the protocol for suspected pneumonia adopted in our ward was applied, and a positive result for the urinary antigen for pneumococcus was obtained. A chest CT scan was performed (◘ Fig. 8.2), which confirmed the presence of extensive parenchymal consolidation of the lingula accompanied by a moderate left pleural effusion.

It was therefore a case of pneumococcal pneumonia with associated parapneumonic pleural effusion, and a correct therapeutic approach was set. The effusion was not abundant, and we had the aetiological diagnosis. Could targeted antibiotic therapy and monitoring of clinical evolution be enough? No!

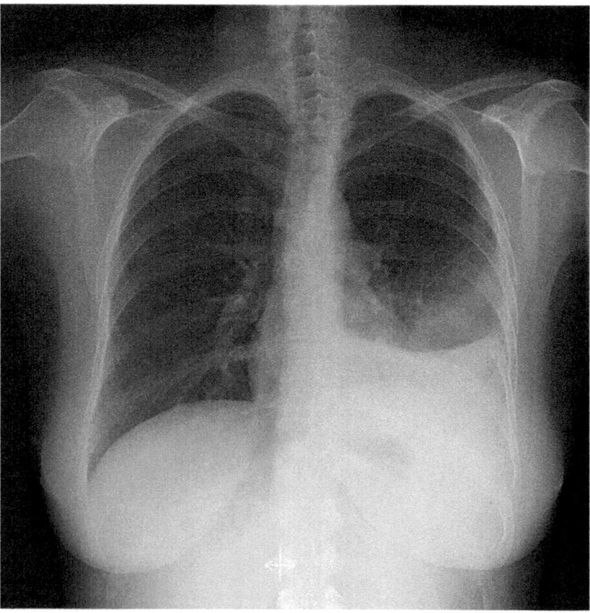

◘ **Fig. 8.1** Chest X-ray at the time of admission

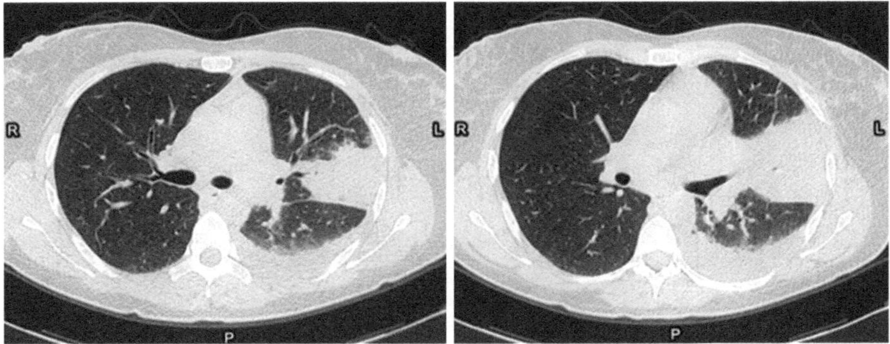

■ **Fig. 8.2** CT of the chest

The correct approach in the case of an infectious pleural effusion should always be to evaluate whether it is a "simple" or a "complicated" effusion [1, 2] (see flow chart in ■ Fig. 8.1 in the chapter on infectious pleural effusion). For this purpose, it is always essential to perform a thoracentesis. An ultrasound of the chest was performed, which documented the absence of loculations and, again under ultrasound guidance, a left posterior thoracentesis was performed which resulted in the aspiration of manifestly purulent pleural fluid with pH = 6. The final diagnosis was therefore pneumococcal pneumonia complicated by pleural empyema. The thoracentesis was interrupted, and a "pig tail" (14-French) thoracic drain was placed, through which around 500 ml of pus were aspirated. Culture examination of the pleural fluid confirmed the presence of Diplococcus Pneumoniae sensitive to piperacillin.

Systemic antibiotic therapy was started with 4 g of piperacillin/0.5 g of tazobactam administered every 8 h; the following day, intrapleural therapy was started with Urokinase 100,000 IU diluted in 100 ml of saline solution for 3 days through the pleural drain. In accordance with the protocol, in the morning, the Urokinase was instilled in the pleural cavity, and the drain was closed for 2 h; it was then reopened and washing with saline solution was performed; lastly, the drain was connected to underwater seal suction with a negative pressure of 20 cmH_2O. Another 600 ml of pus were aspirated.

On the 4th day from the start of therapy, the fever disappeared. After 6 days, at ultrasound, there was no pleural effusion, and no further fluid was drained, and so the drain was removed. The clinical picture rapidly improved, also from the subjective point of view, with the disappearance of the cough. On the 12th day from admission, a chest X-ray was performed (■ Fig. 8.3), and the patient was discharged with a therapy involving amoxicillin/clavulanic acid every 8 h.

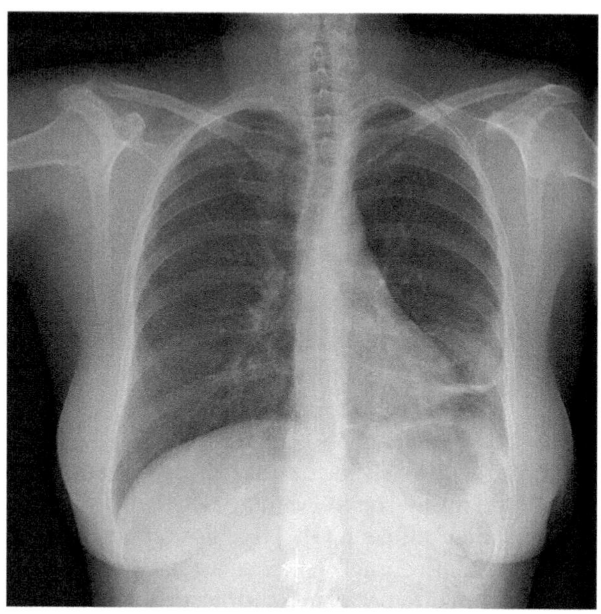

Fig. 8.3 Chest X-ray at discharge

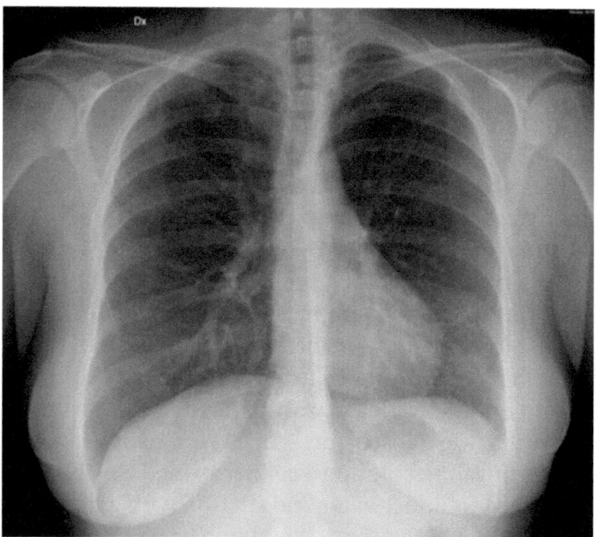

Fig. 8.4 Chest X-ray 1 week after discharge – complete resolution of the radiological picture

A chest X-ray was performed 1 week after discharge (Fig. 8.4), which documented the complete resolution of the radiological picture. Antibiotic therapy was stopped.

We would like to emphasize that no cortisone therapy was performed, since it is useless in these clinical pictures and not recommended by any guidelines! If thoracentesis had not been performed, leading to the correct diagnosis of empyema, the consequent intrapleural medical therapy with fibrinolytic therapy would not have been performed, and the clinical course would have been longer; hence, there would have been an unacceptable negative pleural outcome in a woman as young as 34! Early and correct treatment of pleural empyema avoids the need for surgical therapy.

Conclusive Comments

- Parapneumonic effusion is a common and important complication of pneumonia, which worsens the prognosis.
- It was not a simple pleural effusion but a pleural empyema, and only the prompt thoracentesis followed by the positioning of the drain allowed for a correct diagnostic classification and the consequent treatment.
- Intrapleural therapy with Urokinase, started without delay, allowed for the complete resolution of the clinical-radiological picture.

References

1. Chan KP, Fitzgerald DB, Lee YCG. Emerging concepts in pleural infection. Curr Opin Pulm Med. 2018;24(4):367–73.
2. Dean NC, Griffith PP, Sorensen JS, McCauley L, Jones BE, Lee YC. Pleural effusions at first ED encounter predict worse clinical outcomes in patients with pneumonia. Chest. 2016;149(6):1509–15.

Second Clinical Case of Infectious Pleural Effusion

Loculated Effusion—Thoracoscopic Approach

Angelo G. Casalini

Contents

A. G. Casalini (ed.), *Practical Manual of Pleural Pathology*,
https://doi.org/10.1007/978-3-031-20312-1_9

Here, we present the case history of a 51-year-old male non-smoking labourer, an asthmatic and a diabetic on insulin therapy; 5 days before admission, he developed a high fever (39 °C) and cough. The general practitioner prescribed antibiotic therapy with levofloxacin; in the following days, the patient also presented left chest pain and dyspnoea; the fever persisted and the patient was sent to the emergency department, where a chest X-ray was performed (◘ Fig. 9.1), which highlighted an opacification of the left hemithorax from pleural effusion. The patient was transferred to our ward.

On the patient's admission to our ward, physical chest examination confirmed dullness to percussion with absent fremitus and no breath sounds on the left; urgent blood tests were requested, and a chest CT scan was promptly performed (◘ Fig. 9.2), which documented the presence of a large and loculated left pleural effusion without associated parenchymal lesions. See the flow chart in ◘ Fig. 9.1 in the chapter on infectious pleural effusion.

Haematological tests showed neutrophilic leukocytosis. Antibiotic therapy was initiated with 4 g of piperacillin/0.5 g of tazobactam administered every 8 hours.

The following morning, the patient was taken to the endoscopic room for thoracentesis. An ultrasound of the chest was performed which confirmed the presence of a complex, corpuscular and partially multi-loculated pleural effusion. Under ultrasound guidance, an exploratory puncture was performed with aspiration of pus and the ensuing confirmation of pleural empyema. It was therefore a case of 'primary empyema'. The

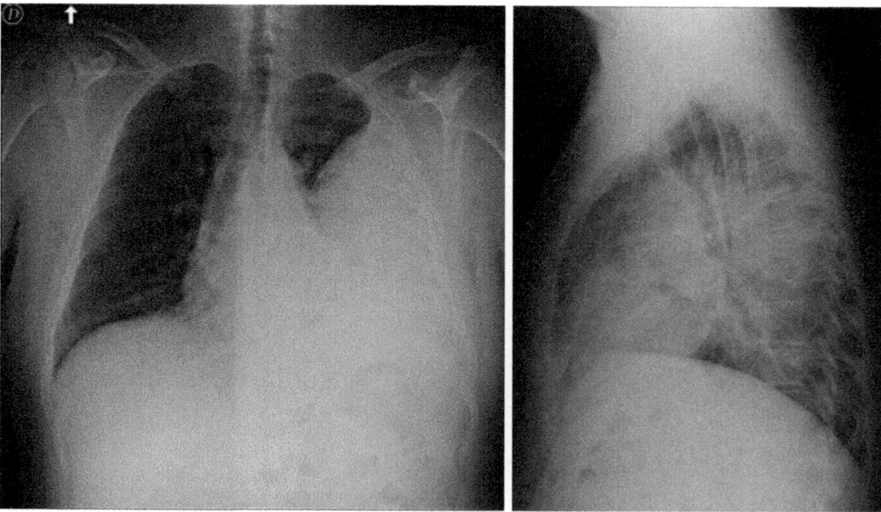

◘ **Fig. 9.1** Chest X-ray at the time of admission to the emergency department

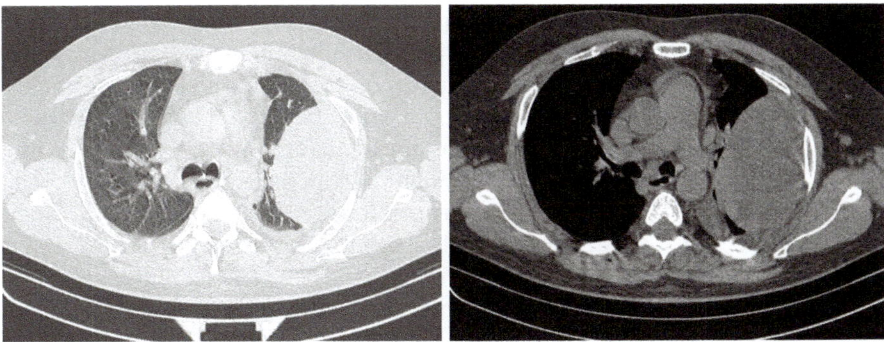

◘ **Fig. 9.2** CT scan of the chest: loculated left pleural effusion

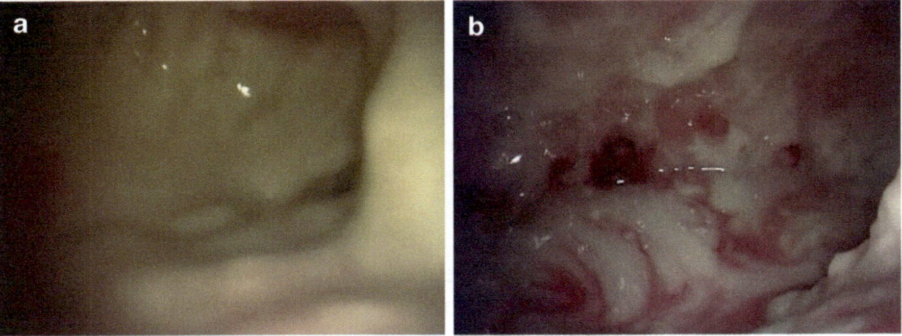

◘ **Fig. 9.3** (**a**) On the left, endoscopic picture at the start of thoracoscopy and (**b**) On the right, after repeated washing with Urokinase and saline solution and aspirations

thoracentesis was interrupted, and we immediately proceeded to a medical thoracoscopy. Medical thoracoscopy was carried out in the endoscopy suite; the patient was placed on his healthy side under local anaesthesia with 2% lidocaine and moderate sedation using midazolam, according to the technique described by Boutin [1] using a rigid 7-mm trocar (Wolf).

The endoscopic picture was characterised by the presence in the pleural cavity of abundant dense pus, which created multiple loculations (◘ Fig. 9.3a). Repeated aspirations and lavages were performed with Urokinase diluted in saline solution, and large clusters of pus were mechanically removed with forceps. These endoscopic manoeuvres took time and patience, but in the end, we obtained a fairly good cleaning of the pleural cavity and were able to explore fairly well the pleural cavity and the parietal pleura, which showed as being markedly thickened, partially covered with a non-removable pus layer and of a clearly inflammatory appearance (◘ Fig. 9.3b). At the end of the cleaning procedure, biopsies of the parietal pleura were performed, which confirmed the diagnosis of suppurative inflammation. Boutin [2] reports that in 1 out of 188 cases of malignant pleural mesothelioma the clinical onset was an empyema, and therefore, the execution of pleural biopsies is always mandatory in these situations. At the end of the examination, the instrument was removed, and a 24-French drain was inserted and connected to underwater seal suction with a negative pressure suction of 20 cm H_2O, and medication was performed. The patient had no complications resulting from thoracoscopy.

The cytological examination of the pleural fluid revealed that it was highly neutrophil-predominant. The microbiological examination of the pleural fluid led to the isolation of *Streptococcus gordonii* sensitive to piperacillin. It is a Gram-positive, facultatively anaerobic bacterium, which belongs to viridans streptococci, and is generally an opportunist frequently present as a saprophyte in the oral flora and may be responsible for bacterial endocarditis [3]. On the basis of this datum, we subjected the patient to an echocardiography, which resulted negative; a dental examination and an orthopantomography were also performed, which were negative.

Since there was no parenchymal involvement, we hypothesised that the pleural infection had occurred by a haematogenous route, although blood culture performed three times was negative. Antibiotic therapy initiated on an empirical basis was confirmed.

Few cases of pleural empyema caused by Streptococcus Gordonii have been reported in the literature [4, 5].

The day after the thoracoscopy, a three-day course of intrapleural therapy with Urokinase 100,000 IU was started, followed each time by washing with saline solution. Since, after the usual three days of therapy in accordance with our protocol, the radiological and ultrasound picture was still not satisfactory, and since with the lavages purulent-looking fluid continued to come out, intrapleural therapy with Urokinase was continued for another 3 days.

On the fourth day from the start of the antibiotic therapy, the patient was completely fever-free. The second cycle of Urokinase therapy was completed.

Fifteen days from admission, the drain was removed and the patient was discharged in excellent clinical condition with the radiological picture below (◘ Fig. 9.4).

At a subsequent clinical follow-up 30 days after the discharge, the patient was well.

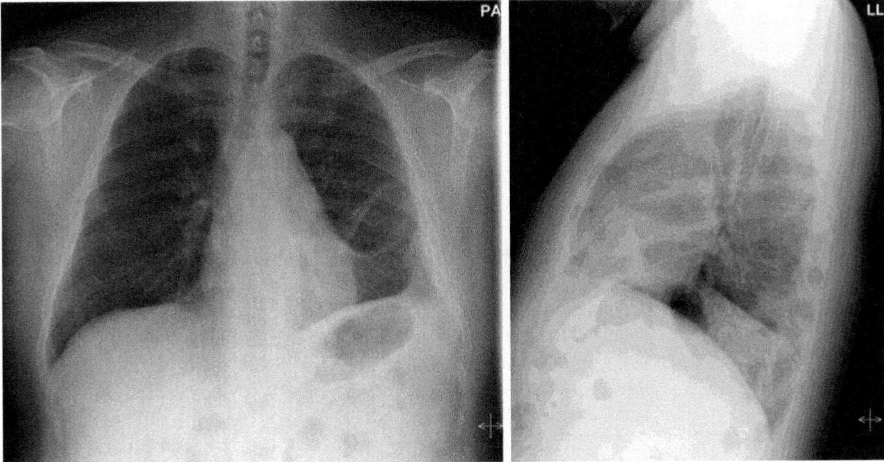

Fig. 9.4 Chest X-ray of the patient at the time of discharge

Conclusive Comments

- The presence of a complicated effusion and/or an empyema requires an urgent therapeutic strategy and a dedicated diagnostic-therapeutic path to be strictly followed.
- The Pulmonologist who manages a patient with infectious pleural effusion must have important skills in the field of Interventional Pulmonology.
- Chest ultrasound is an indispensable tool.
- The presence of multi-loculated effusion at the ultrasound prompted us to perform an immediate Medical Thoracoscopy, which allowed for a good cleaning of the pleural cavity.
- Interventional Pneumology provides all the tools to manage this type of patient correctly; in particular through Medical Thoracoscopy, used without hesitation at the outset, it is possible to successfully treat even severe cases.
- Correct antibiotic therapy is essential! What was the rationale for starting antibiotic treatment with levofloxacin? (See the chapter "Infectious pleural effusion": antibiotic therapy).
- The use of a fibrinolytic associated with pleural washings, preferably used at the initial stages of the empyema, accelerates the resolution of the picture and allows for healing without negative pleural outcomes (e.g. pleural thickening).

References

1. Boutin C, Viallat JR, Aelony Y. Practical thoracoscopy. Berlin: Springer Verlag; 1991.
2. Boutin C, Rey F. Thoracoscopy in pleural malignant mesothelioma: a prospective study of 188 consecutive patients. Part 1: diagnosis. Cancer. 1993;72(2):389–93. https://doi.org/10.1002/1097-0142(19930715)72:2<389::aid-cncr2820720213>3.0.co;2-v. PMID: 8319170.
3. Kilian M, Mikkelsen L, Henrichsen J. Taxonomic study of viridans streptococci: description of Streptococcus gordonii sp. nov. and emended descriptions of Streptococcus sanguis (White and Niven 1946), Streptococcus oralis (Bridge and Sneath 1982), and Streptococcus mitis (Andrewes and Horder 1906). Int J Syst Evol Microbiol. 1989(39):471–84. https://doi.org/10.1099/00207713-39-4-471.
4. Farooq H, Mohammad T, Farooq A, Mohammad Q. Streptococcus gordonii empyema: a rare presentation of Streptococcus gordonii infection. Cureus. 2019;11(5):e4611. https://doi.org/10.7759/cureus.4611. PMID: 31312538; PMCID: PMC6615575.
5. Krantz AM, Ratnaraj F, Velagapudi M, Krishnan M, Gujjula NR, Foral PA, Preheim L. Streptococcus Gordonii empyema: a case report and review of empyema. Cureus. 2017;9(4):e1159. https://doi.org/10.7759/cureus.1159. PMID: 28507831; PMCID: PMC5429153.

Infectious Pleural Effusion

Angelo G. Casalini

Contents

A. G. Casalini (ed.), *Practical Manual of Pleural Pathology*,
https://doi.org/10.1007/978-3-031-20312-1_10

Premise

I was called for a consultation about an elderly patient with pleural effusion and fever. I recommended immediate thoracentesis and possible drainage. My colleague's response was: we usually prescribe antibiotics and cortisone, and if the patient doesn't respond after a week of therapy, we call the Thoracic Surgeon for a drain!

In the previous chapter, two paradigmatic clinical cases of possible and frequent clinical presentations of infectious pleural effusion were presented.

10.1 Introduction

The term 'parapneumonic' should be revised or at least used appropriately

In the context of infectious pleural effusions, it is necessary to distinguish among simple parapneumonic effusion, complicated parapneumonic effusion and pleural empyema. An infectious pleural effusion can be accompanied by a pulmonary infection (pneumonia or lung abscess) and therefore can be a parapneumonic pleural effusion, or present as an entity in its own right and therefore a 'primary empyema' [1]. A recent Australian clinical study published in 2019 showed pneumonia in only 44% (64/164) of community-acquired empyemas and in 22% (88/398) of hospital-acquired empyemas; all were culture-positive pleural infection [2]. In cases that do not have a parenchymal focus, the infection most likely derives from a haematogenous spread. The term 'parapneumonic' is therefore a simplification and should be revised and used only in specific cases!

In this chapter, the points listed in ◘ Table 10.1 will be schematically described and the following flow chart (◘ Fig. 10.1) on the therapeutic approach will be presented and discussed.

Table 10.1 Topics in this chapter

Topics in this chapter	
Entity of the problem	• Incidence and mortality
	• Aetiology
Diagnosis (early)	Imaging:
	• Chest X-ray
	• Ultrasound
	• CT
	Thoracentesis with examinations of the pleural fluid
Therapeutic strategy (early)	• Thoracic drainage
	• Correct antibiotic therapy
	• Supportive therapy
	• Fibrinolytics
	• Medical thoracoscopy
	• Surgery

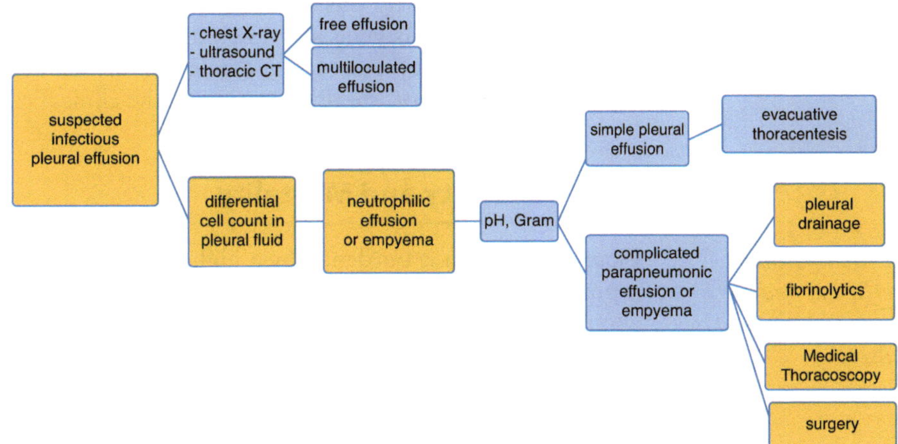

Fig. 10.1 Decisional flow chart on the therapeutic approach to infectious pleural effusion

10.2 Dimension of the Problem and Incidence

In the United States, there are approximately 500,000 to 1,000,000 hospitalisations per year for pneumonia, and about 20% of these are associated with pleural effusions; a complicated effusion or empyema develops in 10% of the effusions [3]. In a more recent Spanish case series [4], out of 4715 patients with CAP, 19% (882) had associated pleural effusions and 30% of these (261) had the characteristics of a complicated pleural effusion or empyema.

The incidence of infectious pleural effusions is increasing

Worldwide, there is an increase in the incidence of infectious pleural effusions and in particular of pleural empyema in adults and children [5–7]. A Finnish study reports more than a doubling of the incidence between the period 2000–2008 and the period 2012–2016, from 4.4 to 9.9 per 100,000 inhabitants and per year [8]. This increased incidence is reported for all aetiologic agents, it is multi-factorial, and its cause is not fully understood. For further information, see the dedicated scientific literature [5–8]. There may be particular risk factors, which can favour the onset of complicated parapneumonic effusion and empyema: poor oral hygiene, chest trauma, drug abuse, alcoholism, diabetes mellitus, abuse or incorrect use of antibiotics. It is important to note that in the first clinical case presented in this manual there were no risk factors, while in the second patient, who was diabetic, a *Streptococcus Gordonii* was isolated, which is generally a coloniser of the oral cavity, an opportunistic pathogen. Please refer to the bibliography reported at the end of the presentation of the clinical case.

10.2.1 Severity and Mortality

Complicated parapneumonic effusion and empyema are burdened by high mortality

Pleural empyema is burdened by a high mortality. Maskell [9] reports a mortality at 1 year of 17% (53/304) in community-acquired empyema and as high as 47% (17/36) in hospital-acquired empyema; the highest mortality rate was for Gram-negative, staphylococcus aureus and mixed infections.

Other authors in a large series of 4424 patients report a mortality at 30 days of 10.8% in community-acquired empyema [10]. According to Colice [11], over 65,000 patients each year in the United States and United Kingdom are affected by infectious pleural effusions, and 15% of these die. A mortality of 15% is also reported in the guidelines of the American Society of Thoracic Surgery [12].

10.2.2 Aetiology

The bacterial aetiology of infectious pleural effusion is different in adults and children and in community-acquired and hospital-acquired infections, and is different from that of pneumonia [13]; this is a fundamental aspect to remember when choosing antibiotic therapy, and therefore, the guidelines for pneumonia should not be a reference [1, 14, 15].

Important studies demonstrating these differences in aetiology are present in the scientific literature and are aimed at identifying the aetiological agents involved. In general, the causative agent is identified in less than 40% to 50% of cases with traditional methods. Molecular investigations improve the diagnostic yield [16, 17]. The use of NAATs (Nucleic Acid Amplification Test) enables us to expand this yield; in Maskell's study [9] the aetiological diagnosis was reached in 74% of cases.

Blood culture is positive in about 14% of patients with pleural infections and may be the only positive aetiological test; it must therefore be performed in all patients [18]. The limited diagnostic yield of the culture test on pleural effusion may depend on previous antibiotic therapies, or on the low concentration of bacteria in the pleural fluid, or on bacteria that are difficult to isolate. The use of a blood culture bottle to collect the pleural fluid directly at the patient's bedside and send it quickly to the laboratory has shown that the yield of the pleural fluid culture increases by about 20% compared to traditional methods [19]. It is important to search for the urinary antigen for Pneumococcus and Legionella. A pleural effusion ranging from 20% to over 60% in the course of Legionella pneumonia has been reported [20, 21].

Different aetiology between community-acquired and hospital-acquired effusions

As previously mentioned, the microbiological tests performed in the MIST1 study [9], a large multi-centre randomised study on infectious effusion with 454 patients recruited, led to the identification of the bacteria responsible in 74% of cases; the results highlight the difference in aetiology between effusions acquired in the community and those acquired in a hospital setting. Among the most frequent bacteria in community-acquired effusions we find the Streptococcus Milleri group [22]; this group includes bacteria responsible for pyogenic infections. The most important characteristic of these bacteria is to cause suppurative infections at various sites, from dental abscesses to abscesses in deep organs. In a study carried out in Canada, Str. Milleri was responsible for half of the cases of empyema [23].

Frequent association with anaerobic bacteria (in 25% of patients)

A very important aspect deriving from the Maskell study and also confirmed by other studies is the high presence of anaerobes, often associated with other micro-organisms in about 25% of community-acquired empyemas; this requires consequent choices in antibiotic therapy (see below). Similar results were also obtained in other studies [24]. In Godfrey's study [25], anaerobes were present in 18% of community-acquired and 11% of hospital-acquired empyemas. In a scientific work that had the main purpose of identifying the presence of anaerobes in 198 patients with pleural empyema [26], anaerobes were identified in 74.2% of cases.

In our experience, which concerns only community-acquired infectious effusions [27], the aetiological diagnosis was obtained in 45/77 (58%) patients and 54 bacteria were isolated, 12 of which were anaerobes; the results are reported in ◘ Table 10.2.

◘ **Table 10.2** Aetiology of infectious effusions in our experience

Isolated bacteria in infectious pleural effusions in our experience	
Streptococci	20 (37%)
• *S. milleri*	8
• *S. pneumoniae*	4
• *S. viridans*	1
• *S. pyogenes*	1
• *S. gordonii* (facultative anaerobe)	1
• Other streptococci	5
Staphylococci	16 (29%)
• *Staph. Epidermidis*	6
• *Staph. Aureus*	4
• *Staph. Hominis*	4
• Other staphylococci	2
Gram-negative aerobes	6 (11%)
• Pseudomonas Aer	2
• Klebsiella Pn.	1
• Enterobatteriacee	3
Anaerobes	12 (22%)
• Fusobacteria	6
• Bacteroides, peptostreptococcus	6

10.3 Diagnosis

The diagnosis of infectious pleural effusion is clinical-radiological, confirmed by thoracentesis. Clinical doubt requires radiological confirmation. Symptoms are: fever (which can also be absent in debilitated subjects), cough, chest pain or dyspnoea; in some patients, there can be a rapid evolution towards a septic state. Already the chest physical examination generally points towards the presence of pleural effusion, but the two indispensable diagnostic moments are the confirmation with imaging and the study of the pleural fluid.

10.3.1 Imaging

Advantages of thoracic ultrasound

Chest X-ray is generally the first investigation performed; the chest ultrasound now available in all pneumology units has many advantages, which will be described in Chap. 18. In summary, they are the possibility of being easily performed at the patient's bedside, the definition of the extent and the possible nature of the effusion and the safe location of the point where to perform the thoracentesis and/or place the thoracic drain. It is possible and advisable to carry out daily monitoring of the evolution of the effusion at the patient's bedside [28]. In many situations, a CT scan of the chest could also be avoided.

10.3.2 Thoracentesis

Thoracentesis: ALWAYS!

In the presence of a pleural effusion of suspected infectious origin (obviously also in the others!), thoracentesis must always be performed! The BTS recommends thoracentesis in all effusions greater than 10 mm [18]. On the other hand, it should not even be necessary to consult the BTS to remember that all effusions must be sampled. Just common sense should be enough and must overcome laziness and a policy of wait-and-see: 'let's see how it goes … we'll do it later'! If the aspirated pleural fluid has a pH ≤ 7.20 or is pus, the manoeuvre must be followed immediately by the placement of a pleural drain; in other cases, an evacuative and not just exploratory thoracentesis is recommended.

It is important to keep smaller effusions under control because it is common to see a rapid increase in pleural fluid in the ensuing hours. Each infectious pleural effusion must be sampled within 24 to 48 h of admission to the hospital.

Thoracentesis provides fundamental and indispensable information to know the characteristics of the liquid, to establish whether it is a simple or complicated effusion and to perform all possible tests: physico-chemical microbiological, cytological examination with differential cell count and pH measurement [29] performed with a blood gas analyser [30]. The pH can be modified by the presence in the syringe of air, heparin or lidocaine and can vary between different locations [31]; however, as recently confirmed, it is an important examination in the evaluation of the patient [32] to distinguish simple from complicated effusions.

Cytological examination of the fluid with the differential count enables us to confirm that the infectious effusion appears as a neutrophilic effusion; however, we must remember that at the initial stages (10–15 days) even the tuberculous effusion is neutrophilic (see the clinical case in the chapter on tuberculous effusion)! Valdés reports that 95% of patients with non-tuberculous infectious pleural effusion had more than 50% of neutrophils in the pleural fluid [33].

10.4 Therapeutic Strategy

Aims:
- *treat the infection*
- *drain the fluid*
- *avoid long-term complications*

The purpose of infectious pleural effusion therapy is to treat the infection and to drain the pleural fluid, allowing the lung to re-expand and thus avoid long-term complications. Therapeutic intervention must be rapid in consideration of the high mortality associated with empyema in particular. High mortality is due not only to the frequent presence of comorbidities, but also to an incorrect and tardy management of the pleural effusion.

The treatment of infectious pleural effusion, and in particular of complicated cases and empyema, cannot be limited to antibiotic therapy alone but must include the points listed in ◘ Table 10.3.

Correct treatment presupposes and derives from knowledge of the evolutive phases (◘ Table 10.4) of the infectious pleural effusion. At the first phase (exudative phase), which lasts about 5–7 days, the pleural effusion is clear, the pH >7.20 and generally the microbiological examination is negative; the subsequent phase (fibrin-purulent phase) is characterised by a drop in pH, which becomes <7.20, by the purulence of the pleural fluid, by the possible formation of loculations, and by the positivity (not always!) of microbiological tests; this phase lasts about another 7 days, and if no action is taken, we move on to the next phase (organising phase) characterised by fibro-

Table 10.3 Therapeutic approach to infectious pleural effusion

Fundamental points in the diagnostic-therapeutic approach to infectious pleural effusion
Correct evaluation with imaging: ultrasound!
Urgent thoracentesis (within 24 h) with execution of all investigations on the pleural fluid
Urgent pleural drainage (within 24 h) in the case of parapneumonic complicated effusion or empyema
Correct antibiotic therapy
Correct treatment of the predisposing factors that favoured the appearance of the clinical picture
Thrombosis prophylaxis with heparin
Intrapleural therapy with fibrinolytics
Medical Thoracoscopy
In particular cases, more invasive surgical procedures

Table 10.4 Developmental phases of infectious pleural effusion

Evolutive stages and treatment of the infectious pleural effusion (parapneumonic or not)			
Stage	**Pleural fluid aspect**	**Pleural fluid characteristics**	**Therapy**
Stage I • Simple parapneumonic effusion	• Yellow	• pH > 7.20 • LDH < 1000 • Glucose >40 mg/dL • Gram: negative	• Evacuative thoracentesis • Antibiotic therapy
• Stage II • (Fibrinopurulent) • Complicated parapneumonic effusion • Empyema	• Yellow (sometimes turbid) • Pus	• pH < 7.20 • LDH >1000 • Glucose <40 mg/dL • Gram: positive	• Pleural drainage • Antibiotic therapy • Fibrinolytics • Medical Thoracoscopy
Stage III • Organising	• Yellow and turbid or pus		• Pleural drainage • Antibiotic therapy • Fibrinolytics • Medical Thoracoscopy • VATS • Surgery

blastic proliferation with thick fibrin membranes that incarcerate the lung. The interval from clinical onset to this phase varies from 2 to 4 weeks; this underlines the importance of early intervention! Too often, we see clinical cases in which only antibiotic therapy is initiated and nothing else is done, except to wait for the outcome of this.

Thoracentesis and the possible placement of a pleural drain must be performed within 48 h of clinical onset

Thoracentesis must always be performed within 48 h of clinical onset at the latest. The delayed diagnostic thoracentesis of an infectious pleural effusion, waiting for a response to antibiotic therapy, is associated with a worse prognosis, longer hospitalisation, increased costs [34] and the presence of negative pleural outcomes. Similarly, a delay of more than 3 days in the placement of the pleural drain after recognition of the effusion is associated with an increase in mortality [35–37].

Thoracentesis and possible very early placement of a drain have the same value as a correct antibiotic therapy!

The previous table (◘ Table 10.4) summarises the evolutionary phases of the infectious pleural effusion with the characteristics of the pleural fluid and the consequent therapies indicated at the respective evolutionary stages.

10.5 Antibiotic Therapy

When choosing the antibiotic, do not refer to the guidelines for pneumonia!

The choice of the correct antibiotic therapy obviously depends on the result of the microbiological tests performed on the pleural fluid. In case of negativity or lack of this data, it is necessary to remember what was previously stated regarding the aetiology, in particular regarding the difference in aetiology between effusions acquired in the community and those acquired in hospital. Maskell [9] points out that in about 50% of community-acquired cases there may be bacteria resistant to penicillin and that in 25% the aetiology includes the presence of anaerobic bacteria. Knowledge of this data is indispensable and indicative in the choice of an empirical therapy.

Important practical advice derives from the BTS [18], to which we refer. The antibiotics that best penetrate the pleural level and which should be the first choice in the case of empirical therapy are penicillins, protected penicillins and cephalosporins. There is indication for metronidazole therapy due to the probable presence of anaerobes. This drug penetrates into the pleural cavity very well. It should be remembered that therapy for anaerobes is not indicated in cases of documented pneumococcal infection and that macrolides are indicated only when there is certainty or strong suspicion of an infection caused by atypical bacteria. Aminoglucosides should be avoided because of their poor penetration into the pleural cavity and because they are inactivated by low pH [38]. There is no indication for intra-pleural instillation of antibiotics. In hospital-acquired empyema, always consider the possible presence of resistant MRSA and Gram-negative bacteria when choosing an empiric antibiotic therapy.

Another aspect to consider is the duration of antibiotic therapy. Some authors [39], in accordance with the BTS guidelines [18], recommend prolonging antibiotic therapy for 3 weeks.

Avoid the use of quinolones in infectious effusions

It is important to remember that the BTS guidelines on the therapy of infectious pleural effusions absolutely do not mention quinolones, although there are scientific papers in the literature that document their good penetration at the pleural level [40, 41].

Migliori [42, 43] warns about the use and abuse of these drugs; since quinolones constitute one of the second-line drugs in the treatment of MDR-TB, there is a potential risk of a selection of quinolone-resistant *M. tuberculosis*.

In our clinical case reported at the beginning of the chapter on pleural tuberculosis, which had been treated with a quinolone, this led to a temporary improvement, followed, however, by distant complications and delayed treatment, as reported in the literature [44]. A recent case report of ours [45] confirms the same problem as to how a 'blind' therapy with a quinolone in a pleural effusion can be responsible for important consequences; for details, see the bibliography.

10.6 Use of Cortisone

In the literature, there is no serious scientific documentation on the use of cortisones

In the literature, and in particular in the most authoritative guidelines, there is no mention of the use of corticosteroids in pleural infections. Only a few experiences in the paediatric field are reported [46], and papers on adults are lacking. The only study—still ongoing, however, at the time of going to print—is a double-blind, randomised controlled multi-centre pilot study on the use of dexamethasone vs. placebo in parapneumonic effusion [47]. See the chapter dedicated to the use of cortisone in pleural pathology.

- *Supportive therapy*
- *Thromboembolic prophylaxis*

Another very important aspect in the management of the patient with infectious pleural effusion consists in supportive therapy ensuring adequate nutritional support, in particular for elderly and debilitated patients. Furthermore, patients with infectious effusion are at high risk of developing thromboembolic disease, and for this reason, with evidence A the BTS [18] recommends heparin prophylaxis.

10.7 Fibrinolytics

The use of fibrinolytics in the pleural cavity is still an open question and divergent opinions exist in the literature. If you do not want to follow only the EBM opinion but also that based on experience, there are several Interventional Pneumology centres, and not only in Italy, where this therapy is regularly adopted with excellent results.

MIST1 [48] was the first multi-centre study to evaluate the efficacy of streptokinase against placebo in the treatment of empyema and complicated parapneumonic effusion and did not show any differences in terms of mortality or the use of surgery. However, a study published in the 2008 Cochrane Review [49], which is recommended reading and which included seven randomised/controlled trials, criticised the Maskell study for its lack of protocol consistency, its use of small-bore drainage tubes and the wide discrepancy in competency of the doctors involved. It should be noted that 52 centres in England were involved, certainly with very different skills despite following the same protocol. The Cochrane Review concluded, however, in favour of a significant reduction in the use of surgery. For further information, see Cochrane [49].

In 2011, the MIST2 study [50] was published which proposes the use of the tissue activator of plasminogen associated with DNase, concluding that it promotes the drainage of pleural fluid, and reduces the use of surgery and the length of hospital stay.

Fibrinolytics used at the beginning of the case play an important role in patient management

A more recent meta-analysis of 2014 [51] on the use of urokinase concluded in favour of a reduction in the need for surgery and a reduction in the length of hospitalisation, without increasing the incidence of severe side effects. A later Cochrane study, from 2019 [52], which includes 12 randomised/controlled trials, partially confirmed the same results; in patients with complicated pleural effusions or empyema, intrapleural therapy with fibrinolytics was associated with a lower percentage of recourse to surgery, without any change in mortality. A recent (2019) article by Porcel [53] concludes that fibrinolytic/DNase therapy removes the need for surgery, and another paper demonstrates that it also appears to be cost-effective [54].

Pleural washing with saline solution is important

From a practical point of view, the drugs usually used are streptokinase (250,000 IU/day for 3 days) and urokinase (100,000 IU/day for 3 days). The drug is introduced into the pleural cavity diluted in 100 mL of saline solution through the drain, which is clamped for about 2 h and then the drop suction is put back on; after a few hours, it is important to associ-

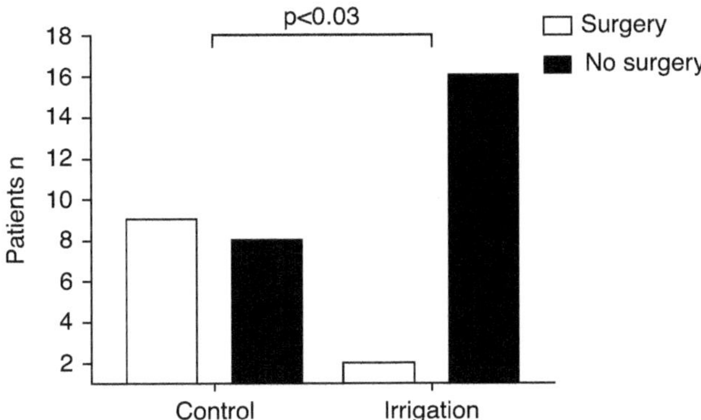

Fig. 10.2 Results of the pleural lavage performed three times a day. (Reproduced with permission of the © ERS 2023: European Respiratory Journal 46 (2) 456–463; DOI: 10.1183/09031936.00147214 Published 31 July 2015 [55])

ate to this method the washing of the pleural cavity with saline solution. The complete treatment can be repeated in case of incomplete or absent response. A manoeuvre that is often underestimated and therefore neglected is that of pleural lavage. In a randomised and controlled study [55], in the group of patients in whom a pleural lavage with saline solution was performed three times a day, the percentage of recourse to surgery was significantly lower (Fig. 10.2). It can therefore be concluded that an inexpensive and simple to implement manoeuvre can contribute to obtaining good results.

The best and officially agreed therapeutic strategy, however, has not yet been established, and much depends on the personal experience and knowledge of the Pulmonologist who manages the complicated pleural effusion and empyema. At the time of writing, a new protocol has been presented, MIST3 [56], which sets this goal. We will see …

10.8 Drainage

Drainage is essential; a drain must be placed immediately!

The placement of a pleural drain is essential in the management of complicated effusion and empyema. Unfortunately, however, this indispensable approach is often delayed or not carried out; the positioning of the pleural drain must always be carried out early in the pleural cavity, preferably under ultrasound guidance. The BTS guidelines [18] absolutely insist on the indispensability of the positioning of the drain in empyema and complicated parapneumonic effusion. The positioning of the drain with aspiration of pus, the use of fibrinolytics and washing of the pleural cavity with sterile saline solution must always be performed before the organisational stage of the effusion is established. Delayed drain placement is associated with increased hospital stay, morbidity, costs and mortality.

In the dedicated chapter, we will mention the various types of thoracic drainage and positioning methods.

10.9 Medical Thoracoscopy

The use of Medical Thoracoscopy is not yet covered by the guidelines, but there are many positive experiences in the literature in favour of this method [57–59]; also in our experience this method has allowed us to achieve excellent results. There is a lack of randomised/controlled trials comparing medical thoracoscopy with other methods. A 1997 randomised/controlled study [60] compared VATS with the use of drainage associated with instillation of streptokinase into the pleural cavity in patients with multi-loculated empyema, and concluded that VATS had superior efficacy (91% success versus 44%), shorter hospital stay and lower costs. Medical Thoracoscopy performed by experienced doctors differs little in results from VATS; this assertion will certainly provoke criticism but is also shared by other Interventional Pulmonologists.

A retrospective study by Brutsche and Tassi [61], in which 127 patients were treated, concluded that in 115/129 (91%) patients, Medical Thoracoscopy had been successful without the need for other interventions. A positive experience was also reported by Ravaglia et al. [62] of 41 patients treated with Medical Thoracoscopy successfully in 91.7% of cases with multi-loculated empyema.

In our experience [27, 63] up to 2012, we treated 77 patients (62 with Medical Thoracoscopy and 15 with pleural drainage) with infectious pleural effusion acquired in the community; 49 of these 77 patients presented with loculated effusions, 16 with organised effusion and 12 with free effusion. We obtained a therapeutic efficacy that did not require further treatment in 73/77 (95%) patients. Only in four patients (two with multi-loculated effusion and two with organised effusion) did we have to turn to the thoracic surgeon; in all these four cases, however, our intervention was unfortunately too late, as the patients had been transferred to us from other departments after 10 to 15 days of hospitalisation in which only antibiotic therapy had been administered! In the 73 patients treated by us, we always performed intrapleural therapy with Urokinase. The results obtained (■ Table 10.5) were the subject of a Specialisation thesis in Pneumology [27].

Table 10.5 Results obtained in our experience in 77 patients

Type of the effusion	Efficacy of the therapy	
	n =	%
Free pleural effusion	12/12	100
Loculated pleural effusion	47/49	96
Organised pleural effusion	14/16	87
Total	73/77	95

Medical Thoracoscopy is an excellent tool to manage the patient with complicated effusion and/or empyema.

It requires specific skills and must be done without delay.

The use of medical thoracoscopy enables us to achieve excellent results even in particularly complex effusions. In the Sumalani et al. study [64], 160 patients who had these characteristics were treated with this method: presence of empyema for over 30 days, lack of response to antibiotic therapy, failure of treatment with pleural drainage, and all multi-loculated empyemas at thoracic ultrasound; there were 102 tuberculous and 58 non-tuberculous empyemas. Medical Thoracoscopy was performed under local anaesthesia in an endoscopic room with a 10 mm thoracoscope. Fibrinolytics were not used. Complete resolution was achieved in 57.5% of patients and partial resolution in 36.25% without the need for further interventions, so medical thoracoscopy was successful in 93.75% of cases. Table 10.6 summarises the results obtained in different experiences with success in 75% to 100% of cases.

A recent Cochrane study [65] considered eight randomised/controlled trials for a total of 391 patients, comparing VATS with chest drainage + fibrinolytics, and concludes there are no significant differences in mortality between surgical and non-surgical treatment; the only advantage of VATS is the reduction in the length of hospitalisation.

This datum also confirms that the discussion remains 'open', and much depends on the local skills involved in the management of this serious disease.

In case of therapeutic failure of drainage or Medical Thoracoscopy, surgical treatment with VATS or thoracotomy with decortication is indicated [66].

Unfortunately, many Pulmonologists consider it easier to entrust the patient to the Thoracic Surgeon and therefore avoid resorting to Interventional Pulmonology, which requires great competence, experience … but also a lot of passion!

One of the most important factors affecting the prognosis of a patient with pleural empyema, in addition to the skills that the Pulmonologist should have, is therefore … to which department he has the good or bad luck to be sent by the emergency department!

Table 10.6 Results obtained with medical thoracoscopy

	Patients treated	Type of study	Pathology	Success %	Surgery %
Solèr 1997 [67]	16	Retrospective	Complicated parapneumonic/empyema	75	25
Brutsche 2005 [61]	127	Retrospective + fibrinolytics	**Multi-loculated**	94	6
Tscheikuna 2009 [68]	12	Retrospective	Empyema	100	0
Ravaglia 2012 [62]	41	Retrospective (23 pts fibrinolytics)	Free flowing 9 **Multi-loculated 24** Organised 8	85.4	14.6
Ali Abo-El-maged 2017 [69]	30	Retrospective	**Multi-loculated**	86.7	13.3
Sumalani 2018 [64]	160	Retrospective	**Multi-loculated**; 30 days after clinical onset	Compl. 57.5 part. 36.25	Not reported
Personal experience 2018 [63]	77	Retrospective + fibrinolytics	Free flowing 12 **Multi-loculated 49** Organised 16	95	5

References

1. Dyrhovden R, Nygaard RM, Patel R, Ulvestad E, Kommedal Ø. The bacterial aetiology of pleural empyema. A descriptive and comparative metagenomic study. Clin Microbiol Infect. 2019;25(8):981–6. https://doi.org/10.1016/j.cmi.2018.11.030. Epub 2018 Dec 21. PMID: 30580031.
2. Brims F, Popowicz N, Rosenstengel A, Hart J, Yogendran A, Read CA, Lee F, Shrestha R, Franke A, Lewis JR, Kay I, Waterer G, Lee YCG. Bacteriology and clinical outcomes of patients with culture-positive pleural infection in Western Australia: a 6-year analysis. Respirology. 2019;24(2):171–8. https://doi.org/10.1111/resp.13395. Epub 2018 Sep 6. PMID: 30187976.
3. Marston BJ, Plouffe JF, File TM Jr, Hackman BA, Salstrom SJ, Lipman HB, Kolczak MS, Breiman RF. Incidence of community-acquired pneumonia requiring hospitalization. Results of a population-based active surveillance Study in Ohio. The Community-Based Pneumonia Incidence Study Group. Arch Intern Med. 1997;157(15):1709–18. PMID: 9250232.
4. Falguera M, Carratalà J, Bielsa S, García-Vidal C, Ruiz-González A, Chica I, Gudiol F, Porcel JM. Predictive factors, microbiology and outcome of patients with parapneumonic effusion. Eur Respir J. 2011;38(5):1173–9. https://doi.org/10.1183/09031936.00000211. Epub 2011 May 12. PMID: 21565916.
5. Burgos J, Falcó V, Pahissa A. The increasing incidence of empyema. Curr Opin Pulm Med. 2013;19(4):350–6. https://doi.org/10.1097/MCP.0b013e3283606ab5. PMID: 23508113.
6. Finley C, Clifton J, Fitzgerald JM, Yee J. Empyema: an increasing concern in Canada. Can Respir J. 2008;15(2):85–9. https://doi.org/10.1155/2008/975312. PMID: 18354748; PMCID: PMC2677840.
7. Nayak R, Lougheed MD, Brogly S, Lajkosz K, Petsikas D. Thoracic empyema - 20 year trends in management and outcomes in Ontario, Canada. Am J Respir Crit Care Med. 2018;197:A4215.
8. Lehtomäki A, Nevalainen R, Ukkonen M, Nieminen J, Laurikka J, Khan J. Trends in the incidence, etiology, treatment, and outcomes of pleural infections in adults over a decade in a Finnish University Hospital. Scand J Surg. 2020;109(2):127–32. https://doi.org/10.1177/1457496919832146. Epub 2019 Feb 21. PMID: 30791827.
9. Maskell NA, Batt S, Hedley EL, Davies CW, Gillespie SH, Davies RJ. The bacteriology of pleural infection by genetic and standard methods and its mortality significance. Am J Respir Crit Care Med. 2006;174(7):817–23. https://doi.org/10.1164/rccm.200601-074OC. Epub 2006 Jul 13. PMID: 16840746.
10. Farjah F, Symons RG, Krishnadasan B, Wood DE, Flum DR. Management of pleural space infections: a population-based analysis. J Thorac Cardiovasc Surg. 2007;133(2):346–51. https://doi.org/10.1016/j.jtcvs.2006.09.038. Epub 2006 Dec 29. PMID: 17258562.
11. Colice GL, Curtis A, Deslauriers J, Heffner J, Light R, Littenberg B, Sahn S, Weinstein RA, Yusen RD. Medical and surgical treatment of parapneumonic effusions : an evidence-based guideline. Chest. 2000;118(4):1158–71. https://doi.org/10.1378/chest.118.4.1158. Erratum in: Chest 2001;119(1):319. PMID: 11035692.
12. Shen KR, Bribriesco A, Crabtree T, Denlinger C, Eby J, Eiken P, Jones DR, Keshavjee S, Maldonado F, Paul S, Kozower B. The American Association for Thoracic Surgery consensus guidelines for the management of empyema. J Thorac Cardiovasc Surg. 2017;153(6):e129–46. https://doi.org/10.1016/j.jtcvs.2017.01.030. Epub 2017 Feb 4. PMID: 28274565.

13. Lisboa T, Waterer GW, Lee YC. Pleural infection: changing bacteriology and its implications. Respirology. 2011;16(4):598–603. https://doi.org/10.1111/j.1440-1843.2011.01964.x. PMID: 21382129.
14. Corcoran JP, Wrightson JM, Belcher E, DeCamp MM, Feller-Kopman D, Rahman NM. Pleural infection: past, present, and future directions. Lancet Respir Med. 2015;3(7):563–77. https://doi.org/10.1016/S2213-2600(15)00185-X. PMID: 26170076.
15. Bedawi EO, Hassan M, McCracken D, Rahman NM. Pleural infection: a closer look at the etiopathogenesis, microbiology and role of antibiotics. Expert Rev Respir Med. 2019;13(4):337–47. https://doi.org/10.1080/17476348.2019.1578212. Epub 2019 Feb 20. PMID: 30707629.
16. Tu CY, Hsu WH, Hsia TC, Chen HJ, Chiu KL, Hang LW, Shih CM. The changing pathogens of complicated parapneumonic effusions or empyemas in a medical intensive care unit. Intensive Care Med. 2006;32(4):570–6. https://doi.org/10.1007/s00134-005-0064-7. Epub 2006. PMID: 16479377.
17. Insa R, Marín M, Martín A, Martín-Rabadán P, Alcalá L, Cercenado E, Calatayud L, Liñares J, Bouza E. Systematic use of universal 16S rRNA gene polymerase chain reaction (PCR) and sequencing for processing pleural effusions improves conventional culture techniques. Medicine (Baltimore). 2012;91(2):103–10. https://doi.org/10.1097/MD.0b013e31824dfdb0. PMID: 22391472.
18. Davies HE, Davies RJ, Davies CW, BTS Pleural Disease Guideline Group. Management of pleural infection in adults: British Thoracic Society Pleural Disease Guideline 2010. Thorax. 2010;65(Suppl 2):ii41–53. https://doi.org/10.1136/thx.2010.137000. PMID: 20696693.
19. Menzies SM, Rahman NM, Wrightson JM, Davies HE, Shorten R, Gillespie SH, Davies CW, Maskell NA, Jeffrey AA, Lee YC, Davies RJ. Blood culture bottle culture of pleural fluid in pleural infection. Thorax. 2011;66(8):658–62. https://doi.org/10.1136/thx.2010.157842. Epub 2011 Apr 1. PMID: 21459855.
20. Pedro-Botet ML, Sabria-Leal M, Haro M, Rubio C, Gimenez G, Sopena N, Tor J. Nosocomial and community-acquired Legionella pneumonia: clinical comparative analysis. Eur Respir J. 1995;8(11):1929–33. https://doi.org/10.1183/09031936.95.08111929. PMID: 8620964.
21. Tan MJ, Tan JS, Hamor RH, File TM Jr, Breiman RF. The radiologic manifestations of Legionnaire's disease. The Ohio Community-Based Pneumonia Incidence Study Group. Chest. 2000;117(2):398–403. https://doi.org/10.1378/chest.117.2.398. PMID: 10669681.
22. Porta G, Rodríguez-Carballeira M, Gómez L, Salavert M, Freixas N, Xercavins M, Garau J. Thoracic infection caused by Streptococcus milleri. Eur Respir J. 1998;12(2):357–62. https://doi.org/10.1183/09031936.98.12020357. PMID: 9727785.
23. Ahmed RA, Marrie TJ, Huang JQ. Thoracic empyema in patients with community-acquired pneumonia. Am J Med. 2006;119(10):877–83. https://doi.org/10.1016/j.amjmed.2006.03.042. PMID: 17000220.
24. Hassan M, Cargill T, Harriss E, Asciak R, Mercer RM, Bedawi EO, McCracken DJ, Psallidas I, Corcoran JP, Rahman NM. The microbiology of pleural infection in adults: a systematic review. Eur Respir J. 2019;54(3):1900542. https://doi.org/10.1183/13993003.00542-2019. PMID: 31248959.
25. Godfrey MS, Bramley KT, Detterbeck F. Medical and surgical management of empyema. Semin Respir Crit Care Med. 2019;40(3):361–74. https://doi.org/10.1055/s-0039-1694699. Epub 2019 Sep 16. PMID: 31525811.
26. Boyanova L, Djambazov V, Gergova G, Iotov D, Petrov D, Osmanliev D, Minchev Z, Mitov I. Anaerobic microbiology in 198 cases of pleural

empyema: a Bulgarian study. Anaerobe. 2004;10(5):261–7. https://doi.org/10.1016/j.anaerobe.2004.06.001. PMID: 16701526.
27. Scarascia A. Infezioni del cavo pleurico. Utilità delle metodiche della Pneumologia Interventistica. Tesi di Specializzazione in Pneumologia. Anno Accademico 2012-13. Università di Parma.
28. Heffner JE, Klein JS, Hampson C. Diagnostic utility and clinical application of imaging for pleural space infections. Chest. 2010;137(2):467–79. https://doi.org/10.1378/chest.08-3002. PMID: 20133295.
29. Sahn SA. Pleural disease. ACCP Pulmonary Medicine Board Review. 25th ed. Glenview, IL: ACCP; 2009. p. 513–46.
30. Rahman NM, Mishra EK, Davies HE, Davies RJ, Lee YC. Clinically important factors influencing the diagnostic measurement of pleural fluid pH and glucose. Am J Respir Crit Care Med. 2008;178(5):483–90. https://doi.org/10.1164/rccm.200801-062OC. Epub 2008 Jun 12. PMID: 18556632; PMCID: PMC2643213.
31. Maskell NA, Gleeson FV, Darby M, Davies RJ. Diagnostically significant variations in pleural fluid pH in loculated parapneumonic effusions. Chest. 2004;126(6):2022–4. https://doi.org/10.1378/chest.126.6.2022. PMID: 15596709.
32. Fitzgerald DB, Leong SL, Budgeon CA, Murray K, Rosenstengal A, Smith NA, Bielsa S, Clive AO, Maskell NA, Porcel JM, Lee YCG. Relationship of pleural fluid pH and glucose: a multi-centre study of 2,971 cases. J Thorac Dis. 2019;11(1):123–30. https://doi.org/10.21037/jtd.2018.12.101. PMID: 30863580; PMCID: PMC6384369.
33. Valdés L, San José ME, Pose A, Gude F, González-Barcala FJ, Alvarez-Dobaño JM, Sahn SA. Diagnosing tuberculous pleural effusion using clinical data and pleural fluid analysis A study of patients less than 40 years-old in an area with a high incidence of tuberculosis. Respir Med. 2010;104(8):1211–7. https://doi.org/10.1016/j.rmed.2010.02.025. Epub 2010 Mar 26. PMID: 20347287.
34. Heffner JE, McDonald J, Barbieri C, Klein J. Management of parapneumonic effusions. An analysis of physician practice patterns. Arch Surg. 1995;130(4):433–8. https://doi.org/10.1001/archsurg.1995.01430040095021. PMID: 7710346.
35. Ashbaugh DG. Empyema thoracis. Factors influencing morbidity and mortality. Chest. 1991;99(5):1162–5. https://doi.org/10.1378/chest.99.5.1162. PMID: 2019172.
36. Sasse S, Nguyen TK, Mulligan M, Wang NS, Mahutte CK, Light RW. The effects of early chest tube placement on empyema resolution. Chest. 1997;111(6):1679–83. https://doi.org/10.1378/chest.111.6.1679. PMID: 9187193.
37. Davies CW, Kearney SE, Gleeson FV, Davies RJ. Predictors of outcome and long-term survival in patients with pleural infection. Am J Respir Crit Care Med. 1999;160(5 Pt 1):1682–7. https://doi.org/10.1164/ajrccm.160.5.9903002. PMID: 10556140.
38. Teixeira LR, Sasse SA, Villarino MA, Nguyen T, Mulligan ME, Light RW. Antibiotic levels in empyemic pleural fluid. Chest. 2000;117(6):1734–9. https://doi.org/10.1378/chest.117.6.1734. PMID: 10858410.
39. Birkenkamp K, O'Horo JC, Kashyap R, Kloesel B, Lahr BD, Daniels CE, Nichols FC III, Baddour LM. Empyema management: a cohort study evaluating antimicrobial therapy. J Infect. 2016;72(5):537–43. https://doi.org/10.1016/j.jinf.2016.02.009. Epub 2016 Mar 15. PMID: 26987740.
40. Chatzika K, Manika K, Kontou P, Pitsiou G, Papakosta D, Zarogoulidis K, Kioumis I. Moxifloxacin pharmacokinetics and pleural fluid penetration in patients with pleural effusion. Antimicrob Agents Chemother.

2014;58(3):1315–9. https://doi.org/10.1128/AAC.02291-13. Epub 2013 Dec 9. PMID: 24323477; PMCID: PMC3957872.

41. Dan M, Torossian K, Weissberg D, Kitzes R. The penetration of ciprofloxacin into bronchial mucosa, lung parenchyma, and pleural tissue after intravenous administration. Eur J Clin Pharmacol. 1993;44(1):101–2. https://doi.org/10.1007/BF00315290. PMID: 8436147.
42. Migliori GB, Langendam MW, D'Ambrosio L, Centis R, Blasi F, Huitric E, Manissero D, van der Werf MJ. Protecting the tuberculosis drug pipeline: stating the case for the rational use of fluoroquinolones. Eur Respir J. 2012;40(4):814–22. https://doi.org/10.1183/09031936.00036812. Epub 2012 May 31. PMID: 22653774; PMCID: PMC3461345.
43. Migliori GB, Zellweger JP, Abubakar I, Ibraim E, Caminero JA, De Vries G, D'Ambrosio L, Centis R, Sotgiu G, Menegale O, Kliiman K, Aksamit T, Cirillo DM, Danilovits M, Dara M, Dheda K, Dinh-Xuan AT, Kluge H, Lange C, Leimane V, Loddenkemper R, Nicod LP, Raviglione MC, Spanevello A, Thomsen VØ, Villar M, Wanlin M, Wedzicha JA, Zumla A, Blasi F, Huitric E, Sandgren A, Manissero D. European union standards for tuberculosis care. Eur Respir J. 2012;39(4):807–19. https://doi.org/10.1183/09031936.00203811. PMID: 22467723; PMCID: PMC3393116.
44. Chen TC, Lu PL, Lin CY, Lin WR, Chen YH. Fluoroquinolones are associated with delayed treatment and resistance in tuberculosis: a systematic review and meta-analysis. Int J Infect Dis. 2011;15(3):e211–6. https://doi.org/10.1016/j.ijid.2010.11.008. Epub 2010 Dec 30. PMID: 21195001.
45. Casalini AG, Cusmano F, Sverzellati N, Mori PA, Majori M. An undiagnosed pleural effusion with surprising consequences. Respir Med Case Rep. 2017;22:53–6. https://doi.org/10.1016/j.rmcr.2017.05.007. PMID: 28702335; PMCID: PMC5487223.
46. Tagarro A, Otheo E, Baquero-Artigao F, Navarro ML, Velasco R, Ruiz M, Penín M, Moreno D, Rojo P, Madero R, CORTEEC Study Group. Dexamethasone for parapneumonic pleural effusion: a randomized, double-blind, clinical trial. J Pediatr. 2017;185:117–123.e6. https://doi.org/10.1016/j.jpeds.2017.02.043. Epub 2017 Mar 28. PMID: 28363363.
47. Fitzgerald DB, Waterer GW, Read CA, Fysh ET, Shrestha R, Stanley C, Muruganandan S, Lan NSH, Popowicz ND, Peddle-McIntyre CJ, Rahman NM, Gan SK, Murray K, Lee YCG. Steroid therapy and outcome of parapneumonic pleural effusions (STOPPE): Study protocol for a multicenter, double-blinded, placebo-controlled randomized clinical trial. Medicine (Baltimore). 2019;98(43):e17397. https://doi.org/10.1097/MD.0000000000017397. PMID: 31651842; PMCID: PMC6824804.
48. Maskell NA, Davies CW, Nunn AJ, Hedley EL, Gleeson FV, Miller R, Gabe R, Rees GL, Peto TE, Woodhead MA, Lane DJ, Darbyshire JH, Davies RJ, First Multicenter Intrapleural Sepsis Trial (MIST1) Group. U.K. Controlled trial of intrapleural streptokinase for pleural infection. N Engl J Med. 2005;352(9):865–74. https://doi.org/10.1056/NEJMoa042473. Erratum in: N Engl J Med. 2005;352(20):2146. PMID: 15745977.
49. Cameron R, Davies HR. Intra-pleural fibrinolytic therapy versus conservative management in the treatment of adult parapneumonic effusions and empyema. Cochrane Database Syst Rev. 2008;(2):CD002312. https://doi.org/10.1002/14651858.CD002312.pub3. Update in: Cochrane Database Syst Rev. 2019;2019(10): PMID: 18425881.
50. Rahman NM, Maskell NA, West A, Teoh R, Arnold A, Mackinlay C, Peckham D, Davies CW, Ali N, Kinnear W, Bentley A, Kahan BC, Wrightson JM, Davies HE, Hooper CE, Lee YC, Hedley EL, Crosthwaite N, Choo L, Helm EJ, Gleeson FV, Nunn AJ, Davies RJ. Intrapleu-

ral use of tissue plasminogen activator and DNase in pleural infection. N Engl J Med. 2011;365(6):518–26. https://doi.org/10.1056/NEJMoa1012740. PMID: 21830966.

51. Nie W, Liu Y, Ye J, Shi L, Shao F, Ying K, Zhang R. Efficacy of intrapleural instillation of fibrinolytics for treating pleural empyema and parapneumonic effusion: a meta-analysis of randomized control trials. Clin Respir J. 2014;8(3):281–91. https://doi.org/10.1111/crj.12068. Epub 2014 Jan 16. PMID: 24428897.
52. Altmann ES, Crossingham I, Wilson S, Davies HR. Intra-pleural fibrinolytic therapy versus placebo, or a different fibrinolytic agent, in the treatment of adult parapneumonic effusions and empyema. Cochrane Database Syst Rev. 2019;2019(10):CD002312. https://doi.org/10.1002/14651858.CD002312.pub4. PMID: 31684683; PMCID: PMC6819355.
53. Porcel JM. Dual intracavitary therapy for pleural infections: leaving reluctance behind. Eur Respir J. 2019;54(2):1901001. https://doi.org/10.1183/13993003.01001-2019. PMID: 31371440.
54. Luengo-Fernandez R, Penz E, Dobson M, Psallidas I, Nunn AJ, Maskell NA, Rahman NM. Cost-effectiveness of intrapleural use of tissue plasminogen activator and DNase in pleural infection: evidence from the MIST2 randomised controlled trial. Eur Respir J. 2019;54(2):1801550. https://doi.org/10.1183/13993003.01550-2018. PMID: 31097519.
55. Hooper CE, Edey AJ, Wallis A, Clive AO, Morley A, White P, Medford AR, Harvey JE, Darby M, Zahan-Evans N, Maskell NA. Pleural irrigation trial (PIT): a randomised controlled trial of pleural irrigation with normal saline versus standard care in patients with pleural infection. Eur Respir J. 2015;46(2):456–63. https://doi.org/10.1183/09031936.00147214. Epub 2015 May 28. PMID: 26022948.
56. Bedawi EO. A randomised controlled trial of the feasibility of early administration of clot-busting medication through a chest tube versus early surgery in pleural infection. ISRCTN registry; 2019. Report No.: ISRCTN18192121. http://www.isrctn.com/ISRCTN18192121. Accessed 3 Jul 2020.
57. Reynard C, Frey JG, Tschopp JM. Thoracoscopie en anesthésie locale dans le traitement des empyèmes: une technique efficace et peu invasive. Med Hyg. 2004;62:2138–43.
58. Tassi GF, Marchetti GP. Il versamento parapneumonico e l'empiema. In: Casalini AG, editor. Pneumologia Interventistica. Milan: Springer; 2007.
59. Tassi GF, Marchetti GP, Aliprandi PL. Advanced medical thoracoscopy. Monaldi Arch Chest Dis. 2011;75:99–101.
60. Wait MA, Sharma S, Hohn J, Dal Nogare A. A randomized trial of empyema therapy. Chest. 1997;111(6):1548–51. https://doi.org/10.1378/chest.111.6.1548. PMID: 9187172.
61. Brutsche MH, Tassi GF, Györik S, Gökcimen M, Renard C, Marchetti GP, Tschopp JM. Treatment of sonographically stratified multiloculated thoracic empyema by medical thoracoscopy. Chest. 2005;128(5):3303–9. https://doi.org/10.1378/chest.128.5.3303. PMID: 16304276.
62. Ravaglia C, Gurioli C, Tomassetti S, Casoni GL, Romagnoli M, Gurioli C, Agnoletti V, Poletti V. Is medical thoracoscopy efficient in the management of multiloculated and organized thoracic empyema? Respiration. 2012;84(3):219–24. https://doi.org/10.1159/000339414. Epub 2012 Jul 24. PMID: 22832393.

63. Casalini AG. Il versamento pleurico infettivo. Rassegna di Patologia dell'Apparato Respiratorio. 2017;32:39–47. https://www.aiporassegna.it/article/view/212.
64. Sumalani KK, Rizvi NA, Asghar A. Role of medical thoracoscopy in the management of multiloculated empyema. BMC Pulm Med. 2018;18(1):179. https://doi.org/10.1186/s12890-018-0745-y. PMID: 30486876; PMCID: PMC6264615.
65. Redden MD, Chin TY, van Driel ML. Surgical versus non-surgical management for pleural empyema. Cochrane Database Syst Rev. 2017;3(3):CD010651. https://doi.org/10.1002/14651858.CD010651.pub2. PMID: 28304084; PMCID: PMC6464687.
66. Scarci M, Abah U, Solli P, Page A, Waller D, van Schil P, Melfi F, Schmid RA, Athanassiadi K, Sousa Uva M, Cardillo G. EACTS expert consensus statement for surgical management of pleural empyema. Eur J Cardiothorac Surg. 2015;48(5):642–53. https://doi.org/10.1093/ejcts/ezv272. Epub 2015 Aug 7. PMID: 26254467.
67. Solèr M, Wyser C, Bolliger CT, Perruchoud AP. Treatment of early parapneumonic empyema by "medical" thoracoscopy. Schweiz Med Wochenschr. 1997;127(42):1748–53. PMID: 9383821.
68. Tscheikuna J, Silairatana S, Sangkeaw S, Nana A. Outcome of medical thoracoscopy. J Med Assoc Thai. 2009;92(Suppl 2):S19-23. PMID: 19562981.
69. Abo-El-maged AHA, Elsamadony MF, El-Shamly MM, Hablas WR. Safety and efficacy of medical thoracoscopy in the management of loculated thoracic empyema. Egyptian J Chest Dis.Tuberc. 2017;66(3):445–51. ISSN 0422-7638. https://doi.org/10.1016/j.ejcdt.2016.12.013.

First Clinical Case of Tuberculous Pleural Effusion

A Young Pregnant Woman

Angelo G. Casalini

Contents

A. G. Casalini (ed.), *Practical Manual of Pleural Pathology*,
https://doi.org/10.1007/978-3-031-20312-1_11

We here report the case of a 26-year-old woman, at 4 months of pregnancy. Her remote pathological history revealed nothing of significance. For about a week, she had had high fever (39 °C), dry cough and left chest pain. She was treated by the General Practitioner with Paracetamol and with unspecified antibiotic therapy. Due to the persistence of the symptoms, she was admitted to our department in March. Physical examination of the chest revealed dullness in the left hemithorax with abolition of the tactile fremitus and absent breath sounds on auscultation.

A chest X-ray was then performed (◘ Fig. 11.1) with adequate protection of the abdomen, which confirmed the presence of a significant left pleural effusion. The blood tests were as follows: red blood cells: 3,880,000 Hb: 10.9, white blood cell count: 6950 (neutrophils: 72%), ESR: 72, D-dimer blood test: 2591 (N.V. 0–245).

A thoracentesis was performed immediately with removal of more than 1 L of intense yellow pleural fluid. A chemical and physical examination was performed with the following results: total protein concentration: 4.1 g/dL (in serum: 5.9), LDH 1101 mg/dL (in serum: 385). A differential cell count of the pleural fluid was performed with the following finding: lymphocytes 61%, eosinophils 38%, polymorphonuclear leukocytes 1%. The pH of the pleural fluid was 7.36.

Empiric antibiotic therapy was started with 4 g of piperacillin/0.5 g of tazobactam every 8 h. The pleural fluid was

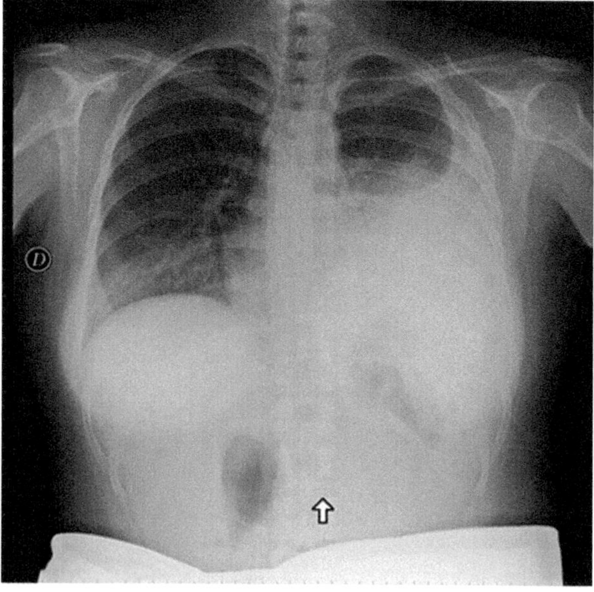

◘ **Fig. 11.1** Chest X-ray performed on admission

sent to the laboratory for complete microbiological investigations: Direct examination did not reveal bacteria and in particular no alcohol acid-resistant bacilli; the Nucleic Acid Amplification Test (TB-NAAT) for *M. tuberculosis* was negative.

After 7 days of therapy, the patient reported reduction in chest pain and decrease in fever (37–37.5 °C); at the physical examination of the chest, left posterior dullness persisted with reduction of the tactile fremitus, for which a second chest X-ray was performed (◘ Fig. 11.2), which demonstrated the persistence of the left effusion, albeit of reduced size.

The ultrasound-guided posterior thoracentesis was repeated, with aspiration of about 100 mL of turbid yellow pleural fluid, which still had the characteristics of the exudate. The differential cell count was repeated with an increase in the lymphocyte component (84%); pH: 7.25. The negativity of the AFB smear and of the TB-NAAT was confirmed in the microbiological examination of the pleural fluid.

In consideration of the marked lymphocytosis of the pleural fluid, the suspicion of tuberculous effusion arose (see the ► Chap. 13) despite the negativity of the microbiological tests, and therefore the need for biopsy confirmation, for which the patient was advised to undergo a medical thoracoscopy. After an adequate explanation of the examination and of its possible side effects, the patient gave her written consent.

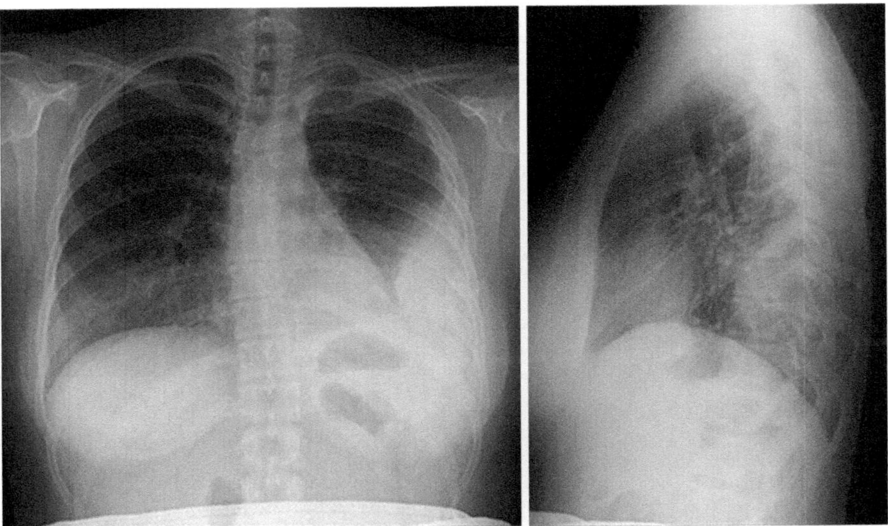

◘ **Fig. 11.2** Chest X-ray performed after 7 days of hospitalisation

On the 12th day after admission, Medical Thoracoscopy, preceded by an ultrasound of the chest, was carried out in the endoscopy suite, with the patient in the lateral decubitus position with the involved hemithorax exposed, under local anaesthesia with 2% lidocaine and moderate sedation using midazolam, in accordance with the technique described by Boutin [1] using a rigid 7-mm trocar (Wolf).

The ultrasound showed the presence of a layer of pleural fluid of about 2 cm sufficient for insertion of the instrument (◘ Fig. 11.3). We then proceeded with local anaesthesia, incision and introduction of the instrument in the left axillary line on ultrasound indication.

During the examination, performed under local anaesthesia and well tolerated by the patient, about 40 mL of manifestly purulent pleural fluid were aspirated; lymphocytes were 97% of the cells present and the pH had dropped to 7.17. After removal of abundant fibrin, only the exploration of a limited portion of the pleural cavity was possible; the parietal pleura, despite the poor quality of the photo, was markedly thickened and hyperaemic (◘ Fig. 11.4). The appearance of the pleural fluid was manifestly purulent with 97% of lymphocytes!

Repeated biopsies and fibrin removals were performed. The day after the thoracoscopy, the results of the microbiological tests performed on the biopsies, on the fibrin and on the pleural fluid arrived, which demonstrated the positivity of both the AFB smear and the PCR. The histological examination also confirmed the diagnosis of tuberculous pleurisy.

The classic anti-tuberculosis therapy was then set up (isoniazid, rifampicin, pyrazinamide, ethambutol for 2 months and then isoniazid and rifampicin for another 4 months), not

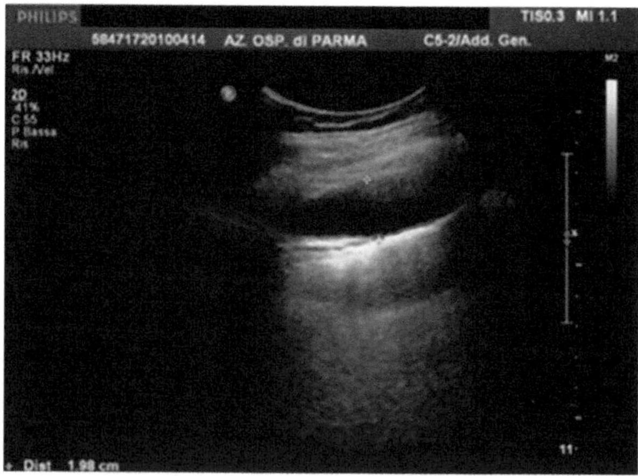

◘ **Fig. 11.3** Chest ultrasound performed before the thoracoscopy

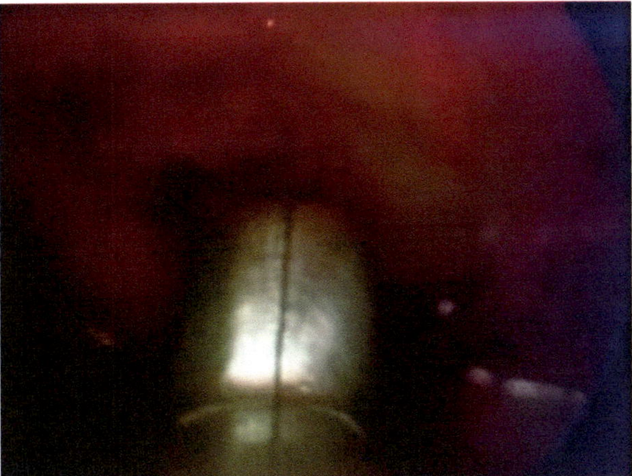

Fig. 11.4 Thickened and hyperaemic parietal pleura with the forceps closed

associated with cortisone therapy. The therapy was carried out until September with regular clinical, ultrasound and laboratory checks, and was shared with the Gynaecologist who was treating the lady. The culture test had shown the lack of resistance to anti-tuberculosis drugs. Anti-tuberculosis drugs can be used safely in pregnancy [2–5]. The clinical course proceeded smoothly without complications, and the end of the therapy coincided with the childbirth, when she gave birth to a beautiful baby!

Conclusive Comments

The clinical case presented lends itself to some comments, in particular regarding the decision taken to perform Medical Thoracoscopy, which made it possible to reach a definite diagnosis, and which in other clinical settings not familiar with the manoeuvres of Interventional Pneumology would not have been taken:

- It was right to include the differential cell count, which demonstrated the lymphocytosis, since, despite the negativity of the microbiological tests, it was this that led to suspected TB.
- Perhaps in other environments, the lymphocytosis would not even have been sought, or else on the evidence of lymphocytosis, an "ex adiuvantibus" therapy would have been undertaken; we have never taken this type of therapy into consideration in other clinical cases, let alone in a pregnant young woman!

- We decided to propose Medical Thoracoscopy to the patient, as the only method that could have clarified the nature of the effusion; the young patient understood the importance of the exam, and accepted it.

References

1. Boutin C, Viallat JR, Aelony Y. Practical thoracoscopy. Berlin: Springer; 1991.
2. Orazulike N, Sharma JB, Sharma S, Umeora OUJ. Tuberculosis (TB) in pregnancy - a review. Eur J Obstet Gynecol Reprod Biol. 2021;259:167–77. https://doi.org/10.1016/j.ejogrb.2021.02.016. Epub 2021 Feb 19. PMID: 33684671.
3. Loto OM, Awowole I. Tuberculosis in pregnancy: a review. J Pregnancy. 2012;2012:379271. https://doi.org/10.1155/2012/379271. Epub 2011 Nov 1. PMID: 22132339; PMCID: PMC3206367.
4. Health Protection Agency. Pregnancy and tuberculosis: guidance for clinicians. London: Health Protection Agency; 2006.
5. Nguyen HT, Pandolfini C, Chiodini P, Bonati M. Tuberculosis care for pregnant women: a systematic review. BMC Infect Dis. 2014;14:617. https://doi.org/10.1186/s12879-014-0617-x. PMID: 25407883; PMCID: PMC4241224.

Second Clinical Case of Tuberculous Pleural Effusion

A 21-Year-Old Man

Angelo G. Casalini

Contents

A. G. Casalini (ed.), *Practical Manual of Pleural Pathology*,
https://doi.org/10.1007/978-3-031-20312-1_12

A 21-year-old man was hospitalised by another department because for about 2 months he had been reporting stinging pain in the left chest and cough; in the previous week, he had presented fever (max 38.5 °C) and general malaise. At the physical examination of the thorax, there was dullness in the lower half of the left thorax with abolition of the tactile fremitus. A chest X-ray was taken (◘ Fig. 12.1), which documented the presence of left pleural effusion. The blood tests were as follows: red blood cells: 5,460,000; Hb: 15.3; white blood cell count: 7500 (N: 67.8%; L: 20.7%; M: 6.2%; E: 3%); ESR: 18; PCR: 33.7; HBsAg positive. Nothing relevant was found in the other blood tests.

Left posterior thoracentesis was performed with aspiration of 1150 cm^3 of pale yellow pleural fluid. It was an exudate with 5.2 g/dL of proteins and with a PF/serum LDH ratio >0.6. Complete microbiological examination of the pleural fluid was performed, with the absence of bacteria; pleural fluid was negative on microscopy for acid-fast organisms and no mycobacteria grew in culture; TB-NAAT was also negative. The cytological examination of the pleural fluid documented lymphocytosis (but the differential cell count was not performed).

After thoracentesis, a CT scan of the chest was performed (◘ Fig. 12.2), which documented a left basal pleural effusion associated with a parenchymal consolidation in the left lower lobe and hilar and mediastinal lymph node calcifications.

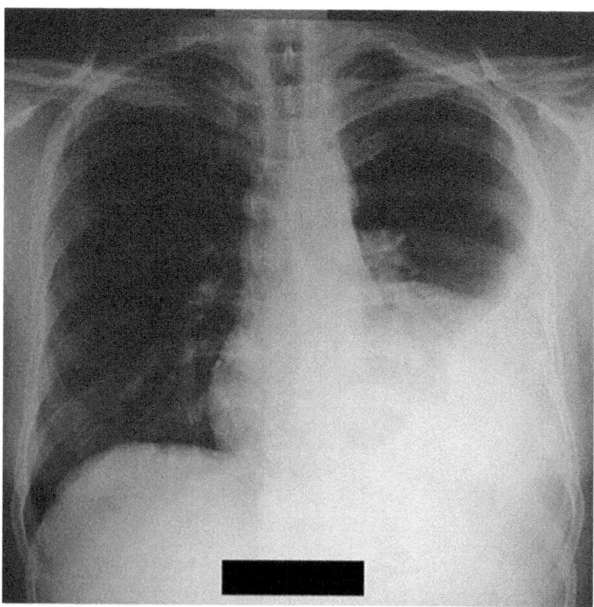

◘ **Fig. 12.1** Chest X-ray at the time of admission

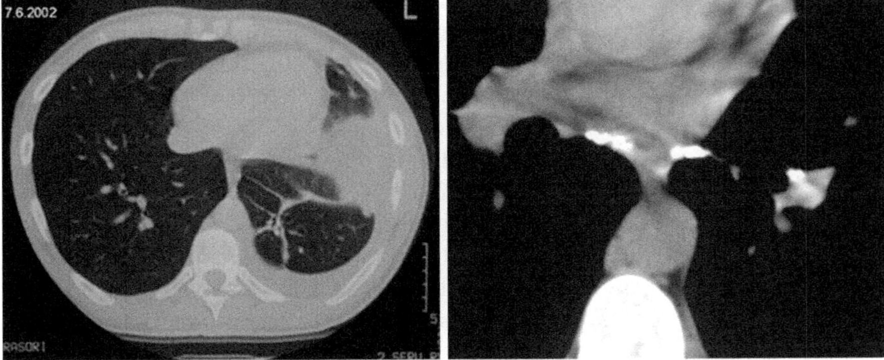

■ **Fig. 12.2** CT scan of the chest

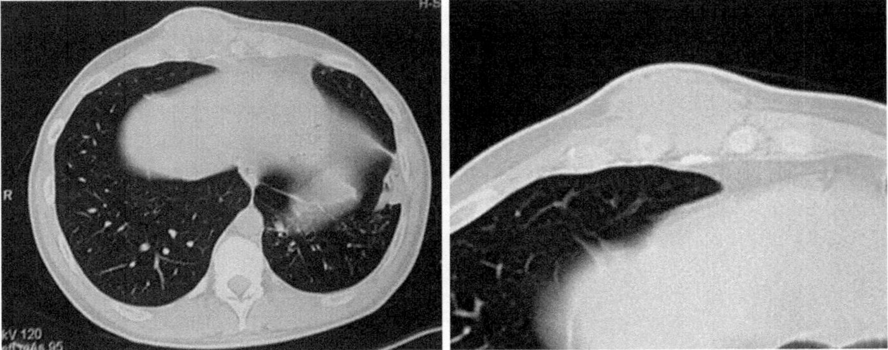

■ **Fig. 12.3** CT scan shows parasternal oval lesion

A normal endoscopic picture was revealed on fibre optic bronchoscopy; selective bronchial washing was performed at the level of the anterior segment of the left basal pyramid for complete microbiological examination including AFB smear, TB-NAAT and culture examination; all investigations were negative.

The following antibiotic therapy was administered: amoxicillin 1 g + clavulanic acid 200 mg IV every 8 h, levofloxacin 500 mg/day per os; complete remission of symptoms was achieved, and the patient was discharged on the 10th day.

The patient was well for 16 months, when finally he came to our department as he presented a painful swelling in the sternal region, without fever. A CT scan of the chest was performed (■ Fig. 12.3), which confirmed the presence of a hypodense oval lesion of the anterior chest wall.

The patient was sent to the surgeon, who under local anaesthesia evacuated and cleaned the abscess formation; the histological examination showed a caseous granulomatous inflammation; the microbiological examination, AFB smear and culture of the aspirated pus were positive for *M. tuberculosis*, without resistance to anti-tuberculous drugs. Skeletal tuberculosis accounts for 1–3% of patients with mycobacterial infection. Any bone can be a site for tuberculosis, although involvement of the sternum is quite rare [1].

In view of the response of the microbiological examination, classic anti-tuberculous therapy was started with four drugs for the first 2 months (rifampicin, isoniazid, ethambutol and pyrazinamide) followed by 4 months of treatment with rifampicin and isoniazid. The symptoms completely resolved with anti-tuberculous therapy.

The topic of infectious pleural effusion therapy is addressed in the ▶ Chaps. 10 and 13. In particular, however, it should be remembered that in the literature it is reported that empirical treatment with fluoroquinolones is associated with a delay in the diagnosis and treatment of tuberculosis [2] and with the risk of developing resistance to quinolones. The "European union standards for tuberculosis care" [3] remind us that, since fluoroquinolones are active against mycobacteria, they can cause a temporary improvement in patients with tuberculosis and should therefore be avoided.

Conclusive Comments

The case report here presented invites various comments, not intended as a criticism of the physicians who followed this patient at the start, but rather as points for serious reflection:

- Too much faith was placed on the negativity of the microbiological examination of the pleural fluid.
- Too little importance was given to lymphocytosis (also without differential cell count) of the pleural fluid.
- The presence of hilar and mediastinal lymph node calcifications in a man as young as 21 should have aroused suspicions.
- In this situation, a medical thoracoscopy would have been diagnostic and would have avoided the subsequent parasternal recurrence.
- Antibiotic therapy with levofloxacin: the BTS 2010 guidelines on infectious pleural effusion do not even include quinolones in the therapy for this type of effusion.

References

1. Cherif E, Ben Hassine L, Boukhris I, Khalfallah N. Sternal tuberculosis in an immunocompetent adult. BMJ Case Rep. 2013;2013:bcr2013008810. https://doi.org/10.1136/bcr-2013-008810. PMID: 23580679; PMCID: PMC3645650.
2. Chen TC, Lu PL, Lin CY, Lin WR, Chen YH. Fluoroquinolones are associated with delayed treatment and resistance in tuberculosis: a systematic review and meta-analysis. Int J Infect Dis. 2011;15(3):e211–6. https://doi.org/10.1016/j.ijid.2010.11.008. Epub 2010 Dec 30. PMID: 21195001.
3. Migliori GB, Zellweger JP, Abubakar I, Ibraim E, Caminero JA, De Vries G, D'Ambrosio L, Centis R, Sotgiu G, Menegale O, Kliiman K, Aksamit T, Cirillo DM, Danilovits M, Dara M, Dheda K, Dinh-Xuan AT, Kluge H, Lange C, Leimane V, Loddenkemper R, Nicod LP, Raviglione MC, Spanevello A, Thomsen VØ, Villar M, Wanlin M, Wedzicha JA, Zumla A, Blasi F, Huitric E, Sandgren A, Manissero D. European union standards for tuberculosis care. Eur Respir J. 2012;39(4):807–19. https://doi.org/10.1183/09031936.00203811. PMID: 22467723; PMCID: PMC3393116.

Tuberculous Pleural Effusion

Angelo G. Casalini

Contents

A. G. Casalini (ed.), *Practical Manual of Pleural Pathology*,
https://doi.org/10.1007/978-3-031-20312-1_13

■■ Premise

I begin this chapter with a curious episode. I had been called for a consultation in a medical department of our hospital for a young male patient with pleural effusion which had started with fever and chest pain. After having visited the patient and seen the clinical documentation, I expressed my hypothesis to my colleague: it's an infectious pleuritis, and it could also be a tuberculous effusion. The colleague asked me an incredible question: and why should he have tuberculosis?

In our experience, 20% of effusions with infectious aetiology were tuberculous.

In the previous chapter, introducing infectious pleural effusions, I reported our experience in which 20% of effusions with infectious aetiology were tuberculous.

Tuberculous pleural effusion accounts for about 25% of cases of extra-pulmonary tuberculosis [1], with a slightly lower incidence than lymph node tuberculosis. The most frequent clinical manifestation is simple tuberculous pleurisy, while tuberculous empyema (◘ Fig. 13.1) is rarer and generally easier to diagnose as it is often associated with parenchymal or bone TB and richer in *M. tuberculosis*.

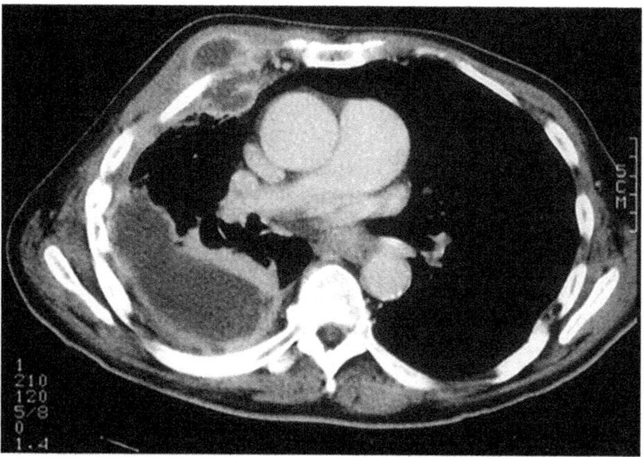

◘ **Fig. 13.1** Right tuberculous empyema associated with bone TB

13.1 Clinical, Laboratory and Radiological Picture

The clinical picture is non-specific and similar to that of other infectious pleurisies.

The clinical picture of tuberculous pleurisy is not indicative and is similar to that of acute infectious pleurisy of other aetiology [2]. The possible tuberculous aetiology must always be evaluated in the face of an infectious effusion, and therefore, it is necessary to strictly follow an adequate diagnostic path. The clinical picture is usually characterised by an acute or subacute onset with fever, cough and chest pain; side symptoms can be night sweats, malaise, weight loss and dyspnoea.

The first investigation that is performed is a chest X-ray, which should always be done in two projections. This is almost always followed by an ultrasonography, which provides further information on the type of effusion and the best place to perform the thoracentesis. The great usefulness of imaging is that it also highlights the possible coexistence of parenchymal lesions and therefore addresses the diagnostic doubt.

The effusion is generally a unilateral lymphocytic exudate, with a low glucose level, and in rare cases can be blood-tinged; it is rarely massive.

The possible presence of concomitant parenchymal lesions is important.

The presence of associated lung lesions varies according to different experiences from 39% [3] to 86% [4]. Therefore, a CT scan of the chest, better if performed after thoracentesis, is crucial to establish if there are parenchymal lesions that are not always clearly evident in a chest X-ray. In our experience, CT scan confirmed parenchymal lesions in 35% (18/52) of patients. The CT scan of ◘ Fig. 13.2 is from a 50-year-old woman with left pleural effusion, who for 30 days had com-

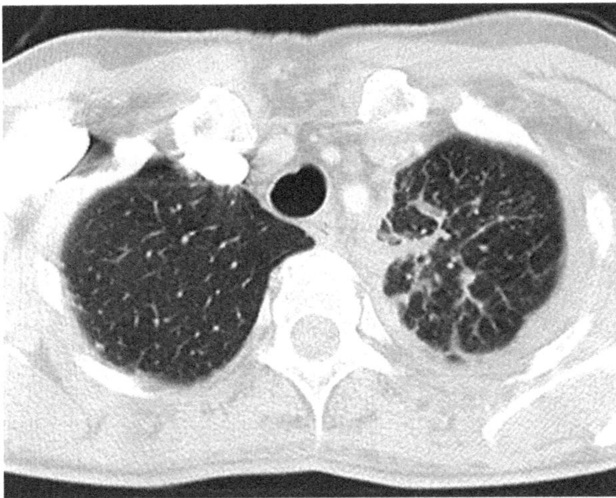

◘ **Fig. 13.2** Micronodulation, ground glass areas and thickened septa in the left upper lobe

plained of cough and fever. Chest X-ray was not conclusive regarding the possible parenchymal involvement; CT scan performed after thoracentesis revealed small non-calcific nodules with ground glass density, thickening of the septa and thickening of the mediastinal pleura in the left upper lobe. The CT picture was considered dubious by the radiologist. The pleural fluid had marked lymphocytosis (97%), and all microbiological tests were negative, including AFB smear and TB-NAAT. A fibre optic bronchoscopy was then performed with selective bronchial lavage in the left upper lobe, which enabled the *M. tuberculosis* to be isolated.

Blood laboratory tests in tuberculous pleurisy are not indicative. Pleural fluid cytology almost always documents lymphocytosis (see below). Mantoux test can be negative in up to 30% of immunocompetent patients [5] and up to 60% of immunocompromised patients.

The markers are only indicative and never diagnostic.

ADA, gamma-interferon and quantiferon have the limitations of not being available in all hospitals and in any case of presenting false negatives and false positives. In Italy, they are not routinely used. ADA in particular, which enjoys extensive use in many countries, depends on the prevalence of tuberculous pleurisy in a certain area; in Italy, where the prevalence is low, the positive predictive value (PPV) is 50% [6]. In any case, the results of these tests cannot be equated with the presence of *M. tuberculosis* in the pleural fluid or in biopsies, and can only be useful if inserted in the correct clinical and radiological context and supported by microbiological data of the pleural fluid and pleural biopsies and by the finding of the histological examination of pleural biopsies. Otherwise, merely on the basis of the positivity of a marker and without a microbiological examination including the important assessment of possible resistance to choose the correct antibiotic therapy, the patient could receive a potentially inefficient therapy with side effects.

BTS Guidelines: tuberculous pleurisy is a treatable cause of lymphocyte effusion (lymphocytes ≥50%).

The BTS guidelines [7] recall that tuberculous pleurisy is a treatable cause of lymphocytic pleural effusion and reiterate the need for a confirmatory pleural biopsy. They also remind us to avoid empirical anti-tuberculous therapy on account of its potential side effects, and to widen the investigations on the pleural fluid and to perform a pleural biopsy to reach a precise diagnosis [7].

13.2 Study of the Pleural Fluid: Importance and Limits

Tuberculous pleural effusion is almost always a lymphocytic effusion. A lymphocytic effusion is also typical of the following situations [8]: neoplastic pleurisy, heart failure effusion, yellow nail syndrome and lymphoma. This means that the presence of a lymphocytic effusion, particularly if associated with clinical signs and symptoms (fever and chest pain) indicative of an infectious effusion, greatly narrows the diagnostic hypotheses.

It is important to perform the differential count of the cells of the pleural fluid.

In the first 15 days, the pleural fluid is 'neutrophilic.'

For this reason, the lymphocytic characteristic of the pleural fluid is an element of great diagnostic importance and, even if not pathognomonic, it can be indicative for hypothesising the tubercular nature of the effusion; this implies that the differential cell count of the pleural effusion should always be made. Valdés [9] reports that in 95% (157/165) of tuberculous effusions, the percentage of lymphocytes was greater than 50%. The pleural effusion is always an exudate and is neutrophilic only at the initial stages (at most in the first 15 days or so), but then there is a change towards lymphocytosis [10]. So there is a neutrophilic tuberculous effusion in the first days and a lymphocytic effusion at the next stage. These two situations give rise to important differences, which it is essential for the physician to know. At the initial phase, the neutrophilic phase, as demonstrated by Bielsa [11], the positive finding of *M. tuberculosis* in the pleural fluid is more frequent than at the subsequent lymphocytic phase (50% compared to 10%).

13.3 Our Experience

In our experience for the diagnostic approach to pleural effusion of suspected tuberculous origin, we used the diagnostic path below (◘ Fig. 13.3), for the details of which we refer to our scientific work [12].

Only the most significant aspects of our case studies are presented below.

There are 52 patients with tuberculous pleural effusion: 20 women (mean age 39 years) and 32 men (mean age 45 years). Twenty-eight out of 52 (53.8%) patients were non-European (most of them from India or Africa). ◘ Figure 13.4 represents the distribution of our patients based on age and provenance. It is clear that the non-European patients were the youngest and that most of the over 60s were Italians.

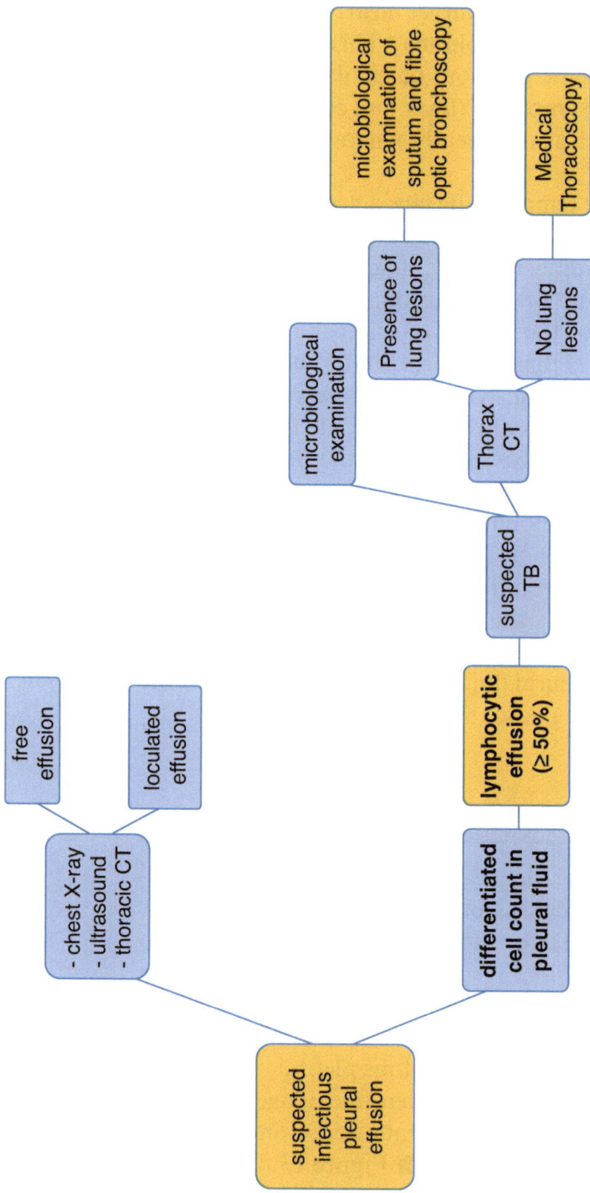

Fig. 13.3 Diagnostic pathway in suspected tuberculous pleural effusion

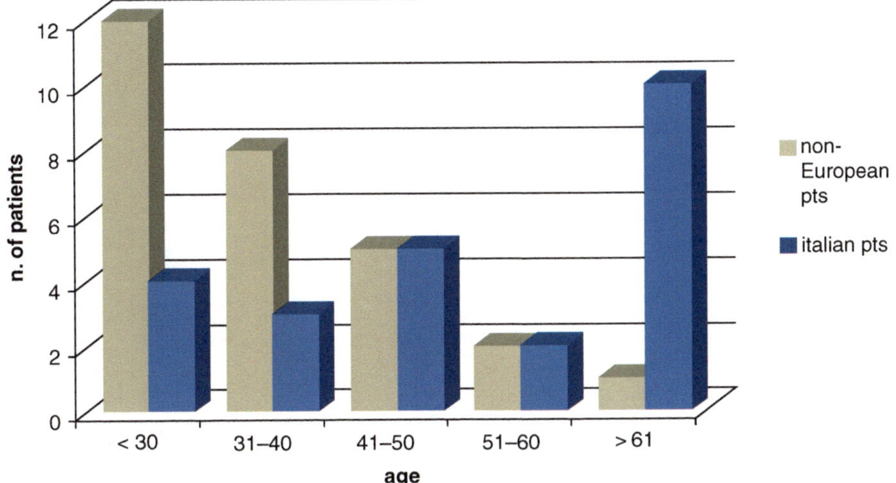

Fig. 13.4 Distribution of our patients based on age and provenance

In 34 patients (65%), there were no parenchymal lesions associated with effusion, while in 18 (35%), there were also pulmonary lesions. In 51/52 patients, there was a lymphocytic effusion (≥50%), and in as many as 44/51 (86%), the percentage of lymphocytes was >85%.

We consider it important to describe the only clinical case in which the effusion was not lymphocytic. This was a 43-year-old Indian male patient. He turned to the emergency room for high fever (39 °C) and acute pain at the base of the right thorax. A chest X-ray (Fig. 13.5) and an abdominal ultrasound were performed; both were negative. The patient was discharged with unspecified antibiotic therapy.

After 3 days, the patient returned to the emergency department because of the persistence of chest pain and fever and the onset of dyspnoea. Chest X-rays and a chest CT scan were done for suspected pulmonary embolism. The presence of embolism was excluded, but right pleural effusion was documented and the patient was hospitalised in our department. A pleural 'pig tail' drain was placed on the right (Fig. 13.6) and 500 mL of yellowish pleural fluid with the characteristics of the exudate were aspirated; differential cell counts documented the presence of 95% neutrophils. A Quantiferon test was also performed, which resulted negative.

The direct microbiological examination and the nucleic acid amplification tests on the pleural fluid were negative, but after 30 days, the positive culture test of pleural fluid for *M. tuberculosis* without resistance to anti-tuberculosis drugs was received. The patient had already been discharged with

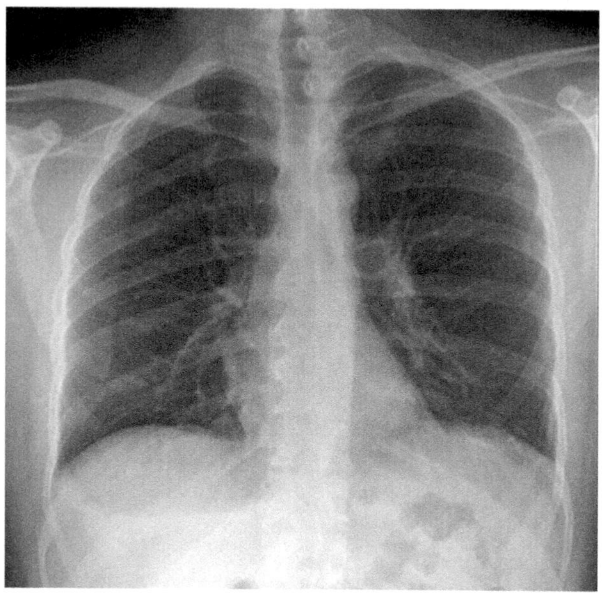

Fig. 13.5 Chest X-ray taken on 29 October

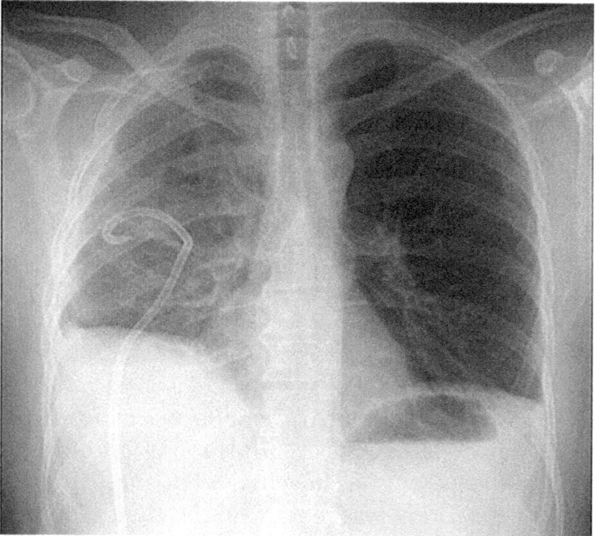

Fig. 13.6 Chest X-ray performed on November 4th after pig tail drain placement

non-specific antibiotic therapy; he was contacted and the classic standard anti-tuberculosis therapy began.

The peculiarity of this clinical case consists in the fact that we had the opportunity to study the patient right at the onset of his clinical history; in fact, at the first access to the emergency room the effusion was not yet present, or at least not evident at chest X-ray! The fact that the effusion was neutrophilic is therefore not a surprise, but in line with what we said previously, namely, that at first the tuberculous pleural effusion is neutrophilic. This was therefore an exception; in usual clinical practice, when one approaches the patient, the 'neutrophilic' phase of the effusion is already over and the effusion is 'lymphocytic'.

Negative correlation between lymphocytosis and positivity of the pleural fluid culture

An interesting scientific work relating to lymphocytosis of the pleural fluid and its clinical importance [13] reports the results obtained on 382 patients affected with tuberculous pleurisy; 83% of these patients had lymphocytosis >55% and, the percentage of lymphocytes was associated with a negative correlation to the probability of obtaining a positive culture test of the pleural fluid.

◻ Table 13.1 shows the results of the microbiological tests on pleural fluid, sputum and bronchoaspirate in our series, and ◻ Table 13.2 shows the results of the microbiological tests on pleural materials.

in 17% of our patients, the culture test on pleural fluid was positive;
in 90% of cases lymphocytosis was present

AFB smear of pleural fluid was positive only in 1/52 patients, TB-NAAT in 8/43 (18.6%) and pleural fluid culture was positive in only 9/52 (17%) patients. These data confirm how misleading it is to consider as significant – as unfortunately so often happens – the negativity of the direct and culture examination of the pleural fluid! So, if we consider that lymphocytosis is present in about 90% of cases and yet the positivity of the culture test is 17%, why is only the microbiological examination usually trusted?

The most suitable materials for diagnosis:
- *pleural biopsy*
- *pleural fibrin*

In our experience, the examination that allowed for the highest diagnostic yield was the pleural biopsy culture, positive in 29/46 (63%) patients. Pleural fibrin is also a very important diagnostic material and must always be collected during thoracoscopy and sent to the microbiology laboratory for a direct and culture examination (positive culture test in 40% of

◻ **Table 13.1** Microbiological results on pleural fluid, sputum and bronchoaspirate

Material	Positive AFB smear	Positive TB NAAT	Positive culture
Pleural fluid	1/52	8/43	9/52 (17%)
Sputum in 11 patients with lung lesions	0/11	0/11	2/11 (18%)
Fibre optic bronchoscopy in 18 patients with lung lesions	2/18	5/18	9/18 (50%)

Table 13.2 Microbiological results on pleural materials

Microbiological results on pleural materials	Diagnostic yield
AFB smear on pleural fluid	1/52 (1.9%)
Culture from pleural fluid	9/52 (17%)
AFB smear from pleural biopsies	3/46 (6.5%)
Culture from pleural biopsies	29/46 (63%)
Culture of pleural fibrin	11/27 (40%)

cases); in one of our patients, we obtained the diagnosis only with a positive fibrin culture test! All patients had a histological picture compatible with tuberculous pleurisy.

It is important to consider the possible coexistence of parenchymal lesions

The result we obtained in the 18 patients with parenchymal lesions is also significant; in 50% (9/18) we obtained a positive culture of *M. tuberculosis* by fibre optic bronchoscopy.

Seven out of the 18 patients with parenchymal lesions had no sputum; we obtained a positive culture of sputum in only two of the remaining 11 (18%). In the literature, a high bacteriological yield (about 50%) on induced sputum is reported even in patients who had pleural effusion, but without parenchymal lesions [14]; therefore, despite having no direct experience, we recommend, when possible, not to neglect this diagnostic possibility.

The M. tuberculosis is in the pleural cavity and must be looked for!

If we compare the results obtained in our series from the culture tests of the pleural fluid and pleural biopsy with those of the literature (Table 13.3), we can see that the yield of the pleural fluid is low, but not the lowest, while the positivity of the pleural biopsy culture stands at the same values as those of the other authors. This means that if *M. tuberculosis* is sought in the pleural cavity it is present in the majority of cases, but it must be sought in the most suitable material, therefore, not only in the fluid, but especially in the pleural tissue!

The initial event in the pathogenesis of tuberculous pleurisy is the rupture of a small sub-pleural caseous focus in the pleural space [15]; mycobacterial antigens enter the pleural space and interact with T cells previously sensitised to mycobacteria; the cause of the effusion is therefore a delayed hypersensitivity response to mycobacterial antigens in the pleural cavity [10].

Quantiferon test was performed in only nine patients and was positive in five (55%); according to our experience, there are no elements to indicate that it is useless, but none to indicate that it is useful!

Table 13.3 Diagnostic yield of microbiological tests on pleural samples (fluid and biopsy)

	Pleural fluid	Pleural biopsy
Berger HW, CHEST 1973 [20]	24%	65%
Epstein DM, CHEST 1987 [21]	35%	47%
Seibert AF, CHEST 1991 [22]	58%	67%
Haro M, Enf Inf Micr Clin 1996 [23]	27%	61%
Kirsch CM, CHEST 1997 [24]	69%	69%
Conde M, AJRCCM 2003 [14]	11%	62%
Diacon A.H. ERJ 2003 [25]	7%	76%
Personal experience [12]	**17.3**	**63%**

A culture test for possible drug resistance is essential!

If we had not performed medical thoracoscopy, the diagnosis would have been made in only 15/52 (28.6%) of the patients; the lack of the results obtained with thoracoscopy would have enabled only a generic diagnosis of 'nonspecific infectious pleurisy' in the remaining patients. So looking into the pleural cavity with the thoracoscopy was similar to opening Pandora's box. In our series, in 4/28 (14%) non-European patients, we isolated resistant mycobacteria: two isoniazid-resistant, one resistant to rifampicin and one MDR-TB. In all four patients, we already had the positivity of TB-NAATs in the pleural fluid. The MDR-TB patient was a young Moldavian woman, 25 years old; she was in the 11th week of pregnancy [16]. She arrived in our ward because of high fever and dyspnoea and with a large left pleural effusion (more than 3 L). Following the appearance of genital bleeding, she underwent a gynaecological examination which documented an internal abortion with 'blighted ovum' [17]. Cytological examination of the pleural fluid with differential counts showed marked lymphocytosis (98.4%). Microbiological tests of the pleural fluid were negative; only TB-NAAT was positive. A medical thoracoscopy was then performed, which showed marked inflammation of the parietal pleura with widespread micronodulation. The microbiological examination on pleural biopsies was positive and led to the isolation of an MDR-*M. tuberculosis*; the histological examination was positive and showed a granulomatous inflammation with necrotising epithelioid and giant cellular cells. Therapy with pyrazinamide, ethambutol, moxifloxacin, linezolid and amikacin was performed with complete resolution of the symptoms.

If we had limited ourselves to the positivity of the TB-NAAT and had started the therapy without performing the thoracoscopy and without the culture obtained on the pleural biopsy, we would have prescribed a useless therapy.

To reiterate the importance of thoracoscopy in the diagnosis of tuberculous pleurisy, a recent work [18] reports the results obtained in various experiences in tuberculous pleurisy with thoracoscopy (◘ Table 13.4). Specificity is 100%, and sensitivity ranges from 90% to 100%.

The endoscopic pictures found in our experience were mainly of two types: at the early stages (◘ Fig. 13.7a) the presence of micronodules in the parietal pleura and, at later stages (◘ Fig. 13.7b), generic signs of marked inflammation in the pleura. The latter was the case of this 40-year-old HIV positive patient, who had had right pleural effusion with dyspnoea and chest pain for several months, and in whom the diagnosis was obtained only through the histological examination of the thoracoscopic pleural biopsy (◘ Fig. 13.8); all microbiological tests (pleural fluid, fibrin and pleural biopsy) were negative.

Some authors also argue the usefulness of blind pleural biopsy with Abrams needle in suspected tuberculous pleurisy as the diagnostic yield is high. In Italy, the method is used only in a few centres. In a study performed on 248 patients with tuberculous pleurisy, the biopsy revealed the typical granulomas in 80% of patients and the biopsy tissue culture was positive in 56% of cases [6]; this particularly high diagnostic yield is explained by the widespread extension of the

Often the endoscopic picture is indicative.

◘ **Table 13.4** Use of medical thoracoscopy in the diagnosis of tuberculous pleurisy. Adapted with permission from Anevlavis 2019 [18]

Study	Patients with TB effusion	Sensitivity	Specificity
Sakuraba (2006) [26]	32	93.8	100
Diacon (2003) [25]	42	100	100
Hansen (1998) [27]	3	100	100
Casalini (2018) [12]	52	100	100
Thomas (2017) [28]	344	90	100
Wang (2015) [29]	333	99	n/a

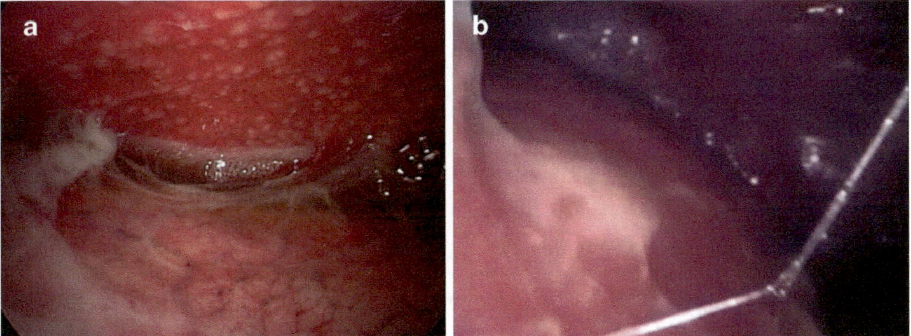

Fig. 13.7 Endoscopic pictures in tuberculous pleurisy; (**a**) early stage (**b**) late stage

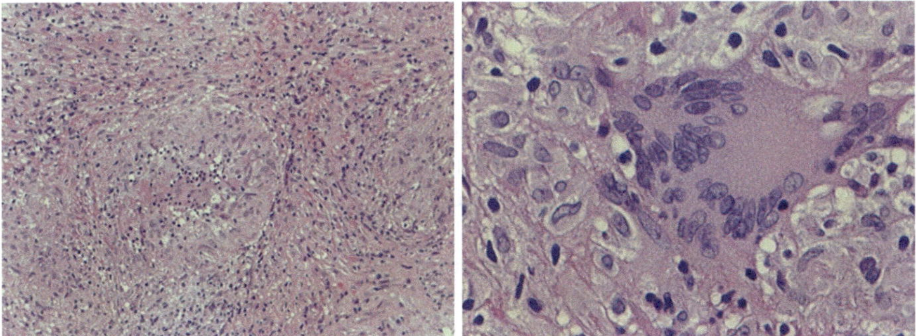

Fig. 13.8 Histological examination of the pleural biopsy

inflammatory process to the parietal pleura; see Fig. 13.3 in the ► Chap. 6.

13.4 Therapy

The therapy for tuberculous pleurisy is the same as for other forms of tuberculosis, and therefore, reference should be made to the literature for therapeutic schemes. As already pointed out, in order to start therapy correctly, it is important to have a culture test available with tests of sensitivity to anti-tuberculous drugs.

It should be noted that no therapeutic scheme of any guideline recommends combining cortisone, and that even a recent Cochrane study [19] does not suggest this therapy since it is useless; the use of cortisone is only recommended for meningeal and pericardial TB.

Table 13.5 Gold standard for the diagnosis of tuberculous pleurisy

Diagnosis of tuberculous pleurisy
By identification of *M. tuberculosis*
1. in pleural fluid
2. in sputum, bronchoaspirate (BAL)
3. in pleural biopsy or pleural fibrin
By pleural histology
1. with blind pleural biopsy
2. with thoracoscopic biopsy

Fundamental role of Interventional Pulmonology and in particular of Medical Thoracoscopy

It can be concluded that the gold standard for the diagnosis of tuberculous pleurisy is therefore the identification of *M. tuberculosis* and/or compatible histological examination (Table 13.5).

The complete diagnostic process for pleural effusion of suspected tuberculous origin cannot be separated from the differential cell count analysis of the pleural fluid and the use of Interventional Pulmonology methods (Fig. 13.3). Medical Thoracoscopy and Fibre optic bronchoscopy, the latter in particular in effusions associated with parenchymal lesions, are indispensable tools. The search for *M. tuberculosis* in pleural fluid rarely leads to the diagnosis, while the presence of lymphocytosis should always be sought as it can be an important guiding element in the diagnosis. In most patients, however, the diagnosis can only be made with pleural biopsy. Tissue is the issue.

13

References

1. Murray JF, Nadel JA. Textbook of respiratory medicine. 2nd ed. Philadelphia, PA: W.B. Saunders; 1994. p. 1094–160.
2. Casalini AG. Il ruolo della toracoscopia nella patologia pleurica tubercolare. In: Casalini AG, editor. Pneumologia Interventistica. Milan: Springer; 2007.
3. Qiu L, Teeter LD, Liu Z, Ma X, Musser JM, Graviss EA. Diagnostic associations between pleural and pulmonary tuberculosis. J Infect. 2006;53(6):377–86. https://doi.org/10.1016/j.jinf.2005.12.023. Epub 2006 Feb 7. PMID: 16466663.
4. Kim HJ, Lee HJ, Kwon SY, Yoon HI, Chung HS, Lee CT, Han SK, Shim YS, Yim JJ. The prevalence of pulmonary parenchymal tubercu-

losis in patients with tuberculous pleuritis. Chest. 2006;129(5):1253–8. https://doi.org/10.1378/chest.129.5.1253. PMID: 16685016.
5. Porcel JM, Vives M. Differentiating tuberculous from malignant pleural effusions: a scoring model. Med Sci Monit. 2003;9(5):CR175-80. PMID: 12761453.
6. Valdés L, Alvarez D, San José E, Penela P, Valle JM, García-Pazos JM, Suárez J, Pose A. Tuberculous pleurisy: a study of 254 patients. Arch Intern Med. 1998;158(18):2017–21. https://doi.org/10.1001/archinte.158.18.2017. PMID: 9778201.
7. Hooper C, Lee YC, Maskell N, BTS Pleural Guideline Group. Investigation of a unilateral pleural effusion in adults: British Thoracic Society Pleural Disease Guideline 2010. Thorax. 2010;65(Suppl. 2):ii4–17. https://doi.org/10.1136/thx.2010.136978. PMID: 20696692.
8. Antony VB, Godbey SW, Kunkel SL, Hott JW, Hartman DL, Burdick MD, Strieter RM. Recruitment of inflammatory cells to the pleural space. Chemotactic cytokines, IL-8, and monocyte chemotactic peptide-1 in human pleural fluids. J Immunol. 1993;151(12):7216–23. PMID: 8258721.
9. Valdés L, San José ME, Pose A, Gude F, González-Barcala FJ, Alvarez-Dobaño JM, Sahn SA. Diagnosing tuberculous pleural effusion using clinical data and pleural fluid analysis A study of patients less than 40 years-old in an area with a high incidence of tuberculosis. Respir Med. 2010;104(8):1211–7. https://doi.org/10.1016/j.rmed.2010.02.025. Epub 2010 Mar 26. PMID: 20347287.
10. Jeon D. Tuberculous pleurisy: an update. Tuberc Respir Dis (Seoul). 2014;76(4):153–9. https://doi.org/10.4046/trd.2014.76.4.153. Epub 2014 Apr 25. PMID: 24851127; PMCID: PMC4021261.
11. Bielsa S, Palma R, Pardina M, Esquerda A, Light RW, Porcel JM. Comparison of polymorphonuclear- and lymphocyte-rich tuberculous pleural effusions. Int J Tuberc Lung Dis. 2013;17(1):85–9. https://doi.org/10.5588/ijtld.12.0236. Epub 2012 Nov 15. PMID: 23164256.
12. Casalini AG, Mori PA, Majori M, Anghinolfi M, Silini EM, Gnetti L, Motta F, Larini S, Montecchini S, Pisi R, Calderaro A. Pleural tuberculosis: medical thoracoscopy greatly increases the diagnostic accuracy. ERJ Open Res. 2018;4(1):00046–2017. https://doi.org/10.1183/23120541.00046-2017. PMID: 29318136; PMCID: PMC5754561.
13. Ruan SY, Chuang YC, Wang JY, Lin JW, Chien JY, Huang CT, Kuo YW, Lee LN, Yu CJ. Revisiting tuberculous pleurisy: pleural fluid characteristics and diagnostic yield of mycobacterial culture in an endemic area. Thorax. 2012;67(9):822–7. https://doi.org/10.1136/thoraxjnl-2011-201363. Epub 2012 Mar 21. PMID: 22436167; PMCID: PMC3426072.
14. Conde MB, Loivos AC, Rezende VM, Soares SL, Mello FC, Reingold AL, Daley CL, Kritski AL. Yield of sputum induction in the diagnosis of pleural tuberculosis. Am J Respir Crit Care Med. 2003;167(5):723–5. https://doi.org/10.1164/rccm.2111019. PMID: 12598215.
15. Stead WW, Eichenholz A, Stauss HK. Operative and pathologic findings in twenty-four patients with syndrome of idiopathic pleurisy with effusion, presumably tuberculous. Am Rev Tuberc. 1955;71(4):473–502. https://doi.org/10.1164/artpd.1955.71.4.473. PMID: 14361964.
16. Majori M, Mori PA, Anghinolfi M, Pisi R, Gnetti L, Motta F, Calderaro A, Casalini AG. Tubercolosi pleurica multir-esistente in gravidanza: challenge diagnostico e terapeutico. Mutidrug-resistent tuberculous pleural effusion in pregnant woman: diagnostic and therapeutic challenge. Rassegna di Patologia dell'Apparato Respiratorio. 2014;29:282–4.

17. Chaudhry K, Tafti D, Siccardi MA. Anembryonic pregnancy. StatPearls. Treasure Island, FL: StatPearls Publishing; 2021. PMID: 29763113.
18. Anevlavis S, Varga C, Nam TH, Man RWC, Demetriou A, Jain N, Lanfranco A, Froudarakis ME. Is there any role for thoracoscopy in the diagnosis of benign pleural effusions. Clin Respir J. 2019;13(2):73–81. https://doi.org/10.1111/crj.12983. PMID: 30578625.
19. Engel ME, Matchaba PT, Volmink J. Corticosteroids for tuberculous pleurisy. Cochrane Database Syst Rev. 2007;(4):CD001876. https://doi.org/10.1002/14651858.CD001876.pub2. Update in: Cochrane Database Syst Rev. 2017;3: CD001876. PMID: 17943759.
20. Berger HW, Mejia E. Tuberculous pleurisy. Chest. 1973;63(1):88–92. https://doi.org/10.1378/chest.63.1.88. PMID: 4630686.
21. Epstein DM, Kline LR, Albelda SM, Miller WT. Tuberculous pleural effusions. Chest. 1987;91(1):106–9. https://doi.org/10.1378/chest.91.1.106. PMID: 3792061.
22. Seibert AF, Haynes J Jr, Middleton R, Bass JB Jr. Tuberculous pleural effusion. Twenty-year experience. Chest. 1991;99(4):883–6. https://doi.org/10.1378/chest.99.4.883. PMID: 1901261.
23. Haro M, Ruiz-Manzano J, Gallego M, Abad J, Manterola JM, Morera J. Tuberculosis pleural: análisis de 105 casos [Pleural tuberculosis: analysis of 105 cases]. Enferm Infecc Microbiol Clin. 1996;14(5):285–9. Spanish. PMID: 8744366.
24. Kirsch CM, Kroe DM, Azzi RL, Jensen WA, Kagawa FT, Wehner JH. The optimal number of pleural biopsy specimens for a diagnosis of tuberculous pleurisy. Chest. 1997;112(3):702–6. https://doi.org/10.1378/chest.112.3.702. PMID: 9315802.
25. Diacon AH, Van de Wal BW, Wyser C, Smedema JP, Bezuidenhout J, Bolliger CT, Walzl G. Diagnostic tools in tuberculous pleurisy: a direct comparative study. Eur Respir J. 2003;22(4):589–91. https://doi.org/10.1183/09031936.03.00017103a. PMID: 14582908.
26. Sakuraba M, Masuda K, Hebisawa A, Sagara Y, Komatsu H. Thoracoscopic pleural biopsy for tuberculous pleurisy under local anesthesia. Ann Thorac Cardiovasc Surg. 2006;12(4):245–8. PMID: 16977293.
27. Hansen M, Faurschou P, Clementsen P. Medical thoracoscopy, results and complications in 146 patients: a retrospective study. Respir Med. 1998;92(2):228–32. https://doi.org/10.1016/s0954-6111(98)90100-7. PMID: 9616517.
28. Thomas, M., Ibrahim, W.H., Raza, T. et al. Medical thoracoscopy for exudative pleural effusion: an eight-year experience from a country with a young population. BMC Pulm Med. 2017;17:151. https://doi.org/10.1186/s12890-017-0499-y.

Wang Z, Xu LL, Wu YB, Wang XJ, Yang Y, Zhang J, Tong ZH, Shi HZ. Diagnostic value and safety of medical thoracoscopy in tuberculous pleural effusion. Respir Med. 2015;109(9):1188–92. https://doi.org/10.1016/j.rmed.2015.06.008. Epub 2015 Jul 3. PMID: 26166016.

13

Exudative Pleural Effusion: Idiopathic Pleural Effusion

Content

Idiopathic Pleural Effusion

Angelo G. Casalini

Contents

A. G. Casalini (ed.), *Practical Manual of Pleural Pathology*,
https://doi.org/10.1007/978-3-031-20312-1_14

Idiopathic pleural effusion is a topic for which, because of the different interpretations and different approaches in managing it, there is no clarity in the scientific literature.

Without claiming to solve the problem, let's try to tackle this topic with the hope of shedding some light and, if possible, even giving some advice!

The diagnostic path of the pleural effusion must be complete!

The diagnostic path of the pleural effusion includes a complete clinical evaluation of the patient with radiological tests, all the indicated laboratory blood tests, all possible investigations on the pleural fluid, and also the use of pleural biopsies, indispensable in many clinical pictures, as in about 25% of cases, the precise diagnosis can only be reached with pleural histology.

Medical Thoracoscopy is certainly the best method of obtaining biopsies on account of its high diagnostic yield and because it usually (in approximately 90%–95% of cases) allows us to successfully complete the diagnostic path. But, even after a careful and complete diagnostic process, a certain number of pleural effusions remain without a definite diagnosis. All of us have happened to be disappointed when a non-orientative histological diagnosis arrived from Pathological Anatomy – from samples on which we had placed all our hopes for a definite diagnosis!

The histological diagnoses we receive in these situations are generic and not indicative: usually non-specific pleuritis, fibrinous pleuritis or pachypleuritis. It is like calling it 'pleuritis X'.

We face a generic histological diagnosis of NSP or similar

A histological diagnosis of 'non-specific pleuritis/fibrosis' (NSP) is defined if the histology report of the pleural tissue revealed any of the following: reactive fibrous pleural thickening, fibrinous pleurisy, fibrosis, florid reactive change, fibrous connective tissue, chronic inflammation, benign change or dense fibrous tissue, in the absence of malignant pleural infiltration, granulomata, pleural vasculitis or evidence of bacterial infection [1].

NSP is a common diagnosis in many benign pathologies

Therefore, although NSP is a detailed and precise definition, it only helps us to exclude, at least temporarily – as in some cases, the patient's follow-up yields some surprises – neoplasms and TB, and is not indicative of other pathologies. In fact, non-specific pleuritis is common to many benign pathologies (also in transudative effusions) [2], the diagnosis of which hinges not only on the histological data but also on a correct diagnostic approach taking into account the clinical context: in effusions associated with drugs or in those associated with connective tissue diseases, or in benign asbestosic effusions and in many other situations.

The incidence of NSP varies in the different experiences from 5% to 30% [2].

It is therefore essential, after completing the diagnostic process, to plan a careful follow-up of the patient, of varying duration in the different clinical experiences, but certainly not less than 1 year [3].

◘ Table 14.1 shows some clinical experiences relating to patients for whom the histological diagnosis of NSP was made and who were followed up over time with follow-ups varying in duration [1, 3–8].

In 5–12.3% of cases of NSP, at follow-up a diagnosis of malignancy emerges, in most cases of mesothelioma

The most important datum that emerges from this table, and from other similar experiences published in the literature, is that in most of these patients during the follow-up (of differing duration) a diagnosis of benign effusion (of different causes) is made or the diagnosis is not reached, and therefore, the effusion is defined as 'idiopathic'. But in a variable percentage, from 5% to 12.3%, the follow-up leads to the diagnosis of malignancy (mainly mesothelioma). The final diagnosis of idiopathic pleuritis was in a percentage of between 25% and 80%.

Table 14.1 Clinical experiences in patients with NSP

Author	Year	NSP	Method of biopsy	No. of malignancies during follow-up	No. of mesothelio-mas	Other diagnoses or lost at the FU	Idiopathic pleuritis	Mean follow-up period (months)
Ferrer	1996	40	Abram's needle	2 (5%)	1	6	32/40 (80%)	62
Venekamp	2005	60	Medical Thoracoscopy	5 (8%)	3/5	40	15/60 (25%)	34.8
Davies	2010	44 (2 excluded)	Medical Thoracoscopy	5 (11%)	5/5	11	26/44 (62%)	21.3
DePew	2014	64	VATS	3 (5%)	3/3	not reported	not reported	60
Gunluo-glu	2015	53	VATS	2 (3.7%)	2/2	24	27/53 (50%)	22.91
Yang	2017	52	Semi-rigid Thoracoscopy	8 (15%)	5/8	23	21/52 (40%)	35.5
Yu	2021	154	Medical Thoracoscopy	19 (12.3%)	6/19	68	67/154 (43%)	61.5

NSP non-specific pleuritis, *VATS* video-assisted thoracic surgery, *FU* follow-up

14.1 When Can We Talk About Idiopathic Pleural Effusion?

Are NSP and idiopathic pleuritis the same? There is discrepancy in the literature; for example, for Reuter [9] the two diagnoses are considered the same. For some authors, the term 'idiopathic' is arbitrarily attributed to a pleural effusion in which repeated cytological examinations of the pleural fluid are negative, for others when the definitive diagnosis is not reached even with pleural biopsies. We believe that the term 'idiopathic pleural effusion' should be used only in cases in which, in addition to the negative pleural biopsies performed by medical thoracoscopy or VATS, an adequate follow-up has been undertaken and a definite diagnosis has not been reached; in reality, therefore, 'idiopathic pleural effusion' does not express a diagnosis, but only our diagnostic 'limits'!

We therefore agree with Wrightson [10]: 'the term "idiopathic pleuritis" is, by definition, a diagnosis of exclusion following exhaustive investigations and judicious follow-up, usually over a period of at least 2 years'.

A 1970 NEJM editorial [11] stated that there seemed to be an agreement to abandon this term, quoting the 1966 issue of Harrison's textbook of internal medicine [12], which said that 'the term 'idiopathic pleural effusion' is idiotic from the standpoint of the physician and pathetic from the standpoint of the patient'. After more than 50 years, however, we are still here talking about idiopathic pleural effusion!

Other definitions – such as cryptogenic effusion, which expresses the lack of knowledge of the aetiology of pleural effusion – have been completely abandoned in the recent scientific literature on pleural pathology; in fact, there is no trace of cryptogenic effusion either in the BTS guidelines [13] or in the latest version of Light's book on Pleural Pathology [14]. The term currently used for a pleural effusion whose cause is unknown is 'idiopathic pleural effusion'.

Therefore, faced with the diagnosis of NSP obtained from histological samples, the most important question is whether it really is a benign effusion or a 'false negative' [2, 15–17]. A false negative can derive from errors in the execution of the biopsy, not performed in sufficient depth (it is necessary to perform a 'biopsy within the biopsy'), or from too limited a number of samples, or from the presence of widespread adhesions that do not allow for the complete exploration of the pleural cavity. In his important book on Practical Thoracoscopy, Boutin recommends taking up to 15 to 20 biopsies of parietal pleura, from widely separate regions of the pleura, including the diaphragm and the costovertebral gutter, even in the case of normal-looking pleura [18].

Some might also think that Medical Thoracoscopy has limits in diagnostics and that VATS instead improves diagnostic yield; however, there is an interesting and recent work by Froudarakis, who compared the diagnostic yield of Medical Thoracoscopy and VATS [17] and concluded that the results were the same.

A careful and personalised follow-up of the patient is important, as suggested by much authoritative literature, especially if there are reasons for suspicion: history of suspected exposure to asbestos, recurrent effusion, doubtful endoscopic picture on thoracoscopy, pleural thickening on CT, fever, weight loss or chest pain. The thoracoscopy must always be repeated in case of suspicion! If the medical thoracoscopy did not allow for the complete exploration of the pleural cavity because of the presence of adhesions, the patient must be sent to the thoracic surgeon for an exploratory thoracotomy!

14.2 Conclusions

- The patient's diagnostic workup must be complete and include pleural biopsies performed with thoracoscopy.
- If a histological diagnosis of NSP or similar is reached, it is important to perform a careful follow-up of the patient (there is no uniformity of behaviour in the literature in the various clinical experiences regarding duration); this follow-up should therefore be personalised for each patient based on age, clinical onset, occupational exposure, possible recurrence of the pleural effusion, possible radiological doubts, etc. [8]. Clinical guidelines recommend close observation of patients with undiagnosed exudative effusions, although the follow-up duration and regime is not defined [19]. In the case of recurrent effusion, the follow-up should include, in addition to clinical checks, the repetition of imaging investigations, laboratory tests and certainly all laboratory investigations on the pleural fluid and, if the diagnosis is not reached, the repetition of the thoracoscopy too.
- There is no justification for the unfortunately common practice of performing *ex adiuvantibus* therapies, e.g., antituberculous therapy or cortisone therapy, without knowing what is being treated.

References

1. Davies HE, Nicholson JE, Rahman NM, Wilkinson EM, Davies RJ, Lee YC. Outcome of patients with nonspecific pleuritis/fibrosis on thoracoscopic pleural biopsies. Eur J Cardiothorac Surg. 2010;38(4):472–7. https://doi.org/10.1016/j.ejcts.2010.01.057. Epub 2010 Mar 12. PMID: 20219385.
2. Janssen J, Maldonado F, Metintas M. What is the significance of non-specific pleuritis? A trick question. Clin Respir J. 2018;12(9):2407–10. https://doi.org/10.1111/crj.12940. PMID: 30004629.
3. DePew ZS, Verma A, Wigle D, Mullon JJ, Nichols FC, Maldonado F. Nonspecific pleuritis: optimal duration of follow-up. Ann Thorac Surg. 2014;97(6):1867–71. https://doi.org/10.1016/j.athoracsur.2014.01.057. Epub 2014 Mar 28. PMID: 24681036.
4. Ferrer JS, Muñoz XG, Orriols RM, Light RW, Morell FB. Evolution of idiopathic pleural effusion: a prospective, long-term follow-up study. Chest. 1996;109(6):1508–13. https://doi.org/10.1378/chest.109.6.1508. PMID: 8769502.
5. Venekamp LN, Velkeniers B, Noppen M. Does 'idiopathic pleuritis' exist? Natural history of non-specific pleuritis diagnosed after thoracoscopy. Respiration. 2005;72(1):74–8. https://doi.org/10.1159/000083404. PMID: 15753638.
6. Gunluoglu G, Olcmen A, Gunluoglu MZ, Dincer I, Sayar A, Camsari G, Yilmaz V, Altin S. Long-term outcome of patients with undiagnosed pleural effusion. Arch Bronconeumol. 2015;51(12):632–6. https://doi.org/10.1016/j.arbres.2014.09.016. English, Spanish. Epub 2015 Jul 26. PMID: 26216715.
7. Yang Y, Wu YB, Wang Z, Wang XJ, Xu LL, Tong ZH, Shi HZ. Long-term outcome of patients with nonspecific pleurisy at medical thoracoscopy. Respir Med. 2017;124:1–5. https://doi.org/10.1016/j.rmed.2017.01.005. Epub 2017 Jan 23. PMID: 28284315.
8. Yu YX, Yang Y, Wu YB, Wang XJ, Xu LL, Wang Z, Wang F, Tong ZH, Shi HZ. An update of the long-term outcome of patients with nonspecific pleurisy at medical thoracoscopy. BMC Pulm Med. 2021;21(1):226. https://doi.org/10.1186/s12890-021-01596-2. PMID: 34253218; PMCID: PMC8276511.
9. Reuter SB, Clementsen PF, Bodtger U. Incidence of malignancy and survival in patients with idiopathic pleuritis. J Thorac Dis. 2019;11(2):386–92. https://doi.org/10.21037/jtd.2018.12.136. PMID: 30962981; PMCID: PMC6409269.
10. Wrightson JM, Davies HE. Outcome of patients with nonspecific pleuritis at thoracoscopy. Curr Opin Pulm Med. 2011;17(4):242–6. https://doi.org/10.1097/MCP.0b013e3283470293. PMID: 21519267.
11. Gaensler EA. "Idiopathic" pleural effusion. N Engl J Med. 1970;283(15):816–7. https://doi.org/10.1056/NEJM197010082831514. PMID: 5456242.
12. Branscomb BV, Harrison TR. Diseases of the pleura, mediastinum, and diaphragm. In: Harrison TR, et al., editors. Principles of internal medicine. 5th ed. New York, NY: McGraw-Hill Book Company; 1966. p. 946–51.
13. Hooper C, Lee YC, Maskell N, BTS Pleural Guideline Group. Investigation of a unilateral pleural effusion in adults: British Thoracic Society Pleural Disease Guideline 2010. Thorax. 2010;65(Suppl. 2):ii4–17. https://doi.org/10.1136/thx.2010.136978. PMID: 20696692.

14. Light RW, Gary Lee YC, editors. Textbook of pleural diseases. 3rd ed. Boca Raton, FL: CRC Press; 2016.
15. Vakil E, Ost D, Vial MR, Stewart J, Sarkiss MG, Morice RC, Casal RF, Eapen GA, Grosu HB. Non-specific pleuritis in patients with active malignancy. Respirology. 2018;23(2):213–9. https://doi.org/10.1111/resp.13187. Epub 2017 Oct 12. PMID: 29024191.
16. Nugent K, Berdine G, Test V. What is the next step in a patient with an undiagnosed exudative pleural effusion? Am J Med Sci. 2020;360(3):211–2. https://doi.org/10.1016/j.amjms.2020.05.009. Epub 2020 May 13. PMID: 32482349.
17. Karpathiou G, Anevlavis S, Tiffet O, Casteillo F, Mobarki M, Mismetti V, Ntolios P, Koulelidis A, Trouillon T, Zadel N, Hathroubi S, Peoćh M, Froudarakis ME. Clinical long-term outcome of non-specific pleuritis (NSP) after surgical or medical thoracoscopy. J Thorac Dis. 2020;12(5):2096–104. https://doi.org/10.21037/jtd-19-3496. PMID: 32642113; PMCID: PMC7330408.
18. Boutin C, Viallat J, Aelony Y. Practical thoracoscopy. 1st ed. Berlin: Springer; 1991.
19. Maskell NA, Butland RJ, Pleural Diseases Group, Standards of Care Committee, British Thoracic Society. BTS guidelines for the investigation of a unilateral pleural effusion in adults. Thorax. 2003;58(Suppl. 2):ii8–17. https://doi.org/10.1136/thorax.58.suppl_2.ii8. PMID: 12728146; PMCID: PMC1766019.

Other Topics

Contents

Pleural Drain: Clinical Case of Pleural Effusion Treated with Small-Bore Pleural Drain

P. A. Mori

Contents

A. G. Casalini (ed.), *Practical Manual of Pleural Pathology*,
https://doi.org/10.1007/978-3-031-20312-1_15

Here, we present the case history of an 85-year-old male ex-smoker affected by COPD and secondary pulmonary hypertension, admitted to the emergency department for severe acute respiratory failure. At admission, the patient was afebrile, tachycardic (heart rate 110 bpm) and tachypneic (respiratory rate 34 bpm). Arterial blood gas analysis revealed a pH of 7.35, a partial carbon dioxide pressure ($PaCO_2$) of 65 mmHg, a partial oxygen pressure (PaO_2) of 59.5 mmHg and an oxygen saturation (SO_2) of 86% with oxygen supplementation. Non-invasive ventilation was started, with 0.6 FiO_2, 7 cm H_2O support pressure (SP), and 10 cm H_2O positive end expiratory pressure (PEEP).

A chest X-ray (◘ Fig. 15.1) revealed an opacification of the left hemithorax from pleural effusion. A chest CT confirmed the presence of two left loculated pleural effusions (◘ Fig. 15.2).

After thoracic ultrasound (TUS) (which diagnosed complex non-septated pleural effusion), a bedside thoracentesis was performed in the intensive respiratory unit, yielding foul-smelling pus. We immediately positioned a Seldinger Cook 14 F chest drain [1]. We could argue about the use of a small-bore chest tube for empyema, but in a situation of urgency at the bedside of the patient, it undoubtedly has some advantages, being a quick and safe procedure [2].

We started with 100,000 IU Urokinase for 5 days. Furthermore, every day regular flushes with saline solution were done to maintain the patency of the small-bore catheter.

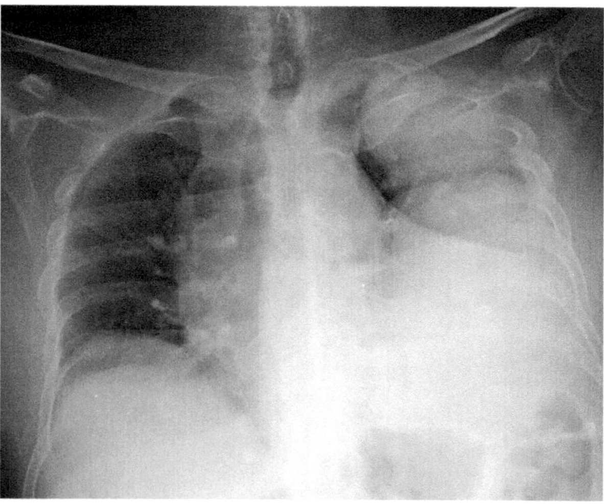

◘ **Fig. 15.1** Chest X-ray at the time of admission to the emergency department

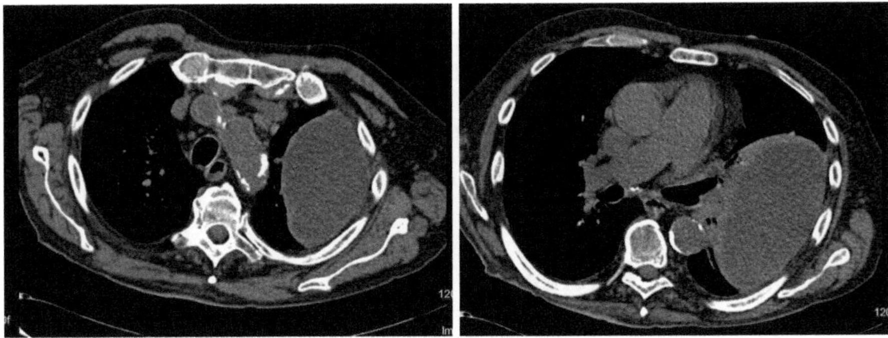

Fig. 15.2 CT scan of the chest: loculated left pleural effusion

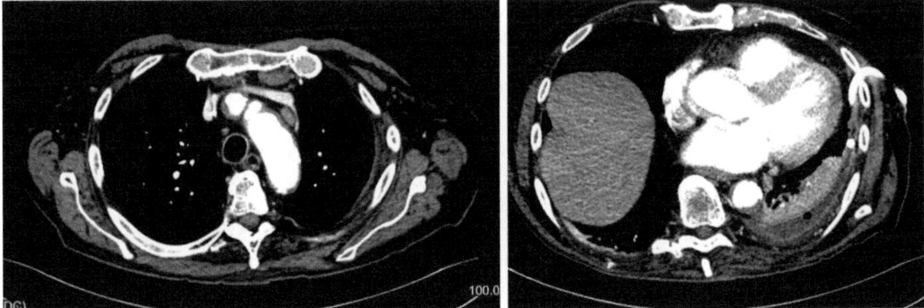

Fig. 15.3 CT scan after 2 weeks

At the same time, an antibiotic therapy was initiated with 4 g of piperacillin/0.5 g of tazobactam administered every 8 h and 500 mg metronidazole every 12 h [3].

The microbiological examination of the pleural fluid was negative, but that is usual in a high percentage of complicated pleural infections, up to 40% [4].

After 10 days, the drainage was removed and a CT scan was done, which showed the excellent clinical course of the pleural infection (Fig. 15.3).

Conclusive Comments

- The presence of an effusion requires an immediate therapeutic strategy.
- Prompt intervention is really important if the patient is in a dangerous clinical situation.
- Thoracic ultrasound is an indispensable bedside tool.
- The size and type of pleural drain is an important decision, to be taken by the pulmonologist.

- The use of a small-bore chest drain inserted with the Seldinger method is a less invasive technique than the trocar method and with practice is a quick and safe procedure.
- The smaller-bore tubes may be the initial treatment of choice for pleural infection.

References

1. Hallifax RJ, Psallidas I, Rahman NM. Chest drain size: the debate continues. Curr Pulmo Rep. 2017;6(1):26–9. https://doi.org/10.1007/s13665-017-0162-3. Epub 2017 Jan 26. PMID: 28344925; PMCID: PMC5346594.
2. Rahman NM, Maskell NA, Davies CW, Hedley EL, Nunn AJ, Gleeson FV, Davies RJ. The relationship between chest tube size and clinical outcome in pleural infection. Chest. 2010;137(3):536–43. https://doi.org/10.1378/chest.09-1044. Epub 2009 Oct 9. PMID: 19820073.
3. Koppurapu V, Meena N. A review of the management of complex parapneumonic effusion in adults. J Thorac Dis. 2017;9(7):2135–41. https://doi.org/10.21037/jtd.2017.06.21. PMID: 28840015; PMCID: PMC5542983.
4. Ferreiro L, San José ME, Valdés L. Management of parapneumonic pleural effusion in adults. Arch Bronconeumol. 2015;51(12):637–46. https://doi.org/10.1016/j.arbres.2015.01.009. English, Spanish. Epub 2015 Mar 26. PMID: 25820035.

Chest Tube Drainage

P. A. Mori

Contents

A. G. Casalini (ed.), *Practical Manual of Pleural Pathology*,
https://doi.org/10.1007/978-3-031-20312-1_16

A chest drain is by definition a flexible tube that is inserted through the ribs into the pleural space.

The drains can vary in size from 6 to 40 F. Most are fenestrated to allow for a better outflow of air or fluid and contain a radio-opaque strip to identify them radiographically. The chest drain must be considered as part of a system that also includes an aspiration system to which the drain itself must be connected to allow for the collection of air or fluid. This aspiration system and its management are of equal importance to the positioning of the drain.

16.1 Indications

The pleural drain serves to create a negative pressure in the pleural cavity and the resulting re-expansion of the lung by removing air or fluid. The main indications [1] are listed in ◘ Table 16.1.

◘ **Table 16.1** Indications for chest drain placement
Pneumothorax
Pleural effusion:
• complicated parapneumonic effusion and empyema
• symptomatic malignant effusion
• benign symptomatic pleural effusion (heart failure, renal failure, cirrhosis) considering the risk–benefit ratio in frail patients
• refractory effusion (especially neoplastic) to perform pleurodesis
• haemothorax
• chylothorax
• postoperative after thoracoscopy or thoracic, cardiac and oesophageal surgery

16.2 Contraindications

There are no absolute contraindications to the placement of a drain other than the absence of a useful pleural space, for example due to the presence of secondary adhesions to previous surgery, lung infections or trauma. Relative contraindications can be the presence of coagulation pathologies or diaphragmatic hernias.

There are no absolute contraindications.

16.3 Patient Preparation

A chest X-ray and often a chest CT scan are usually performed before placing a chest drain. But the most important change in the practice of interventional pneumology, particularly in the placement of a drain, is the general adoption of Thoracic Ultrasound (TUS). The scan (which is done in a quick and safe way at the patient's bedside or in the endoscopic room) enables us to confirm the indication for the procedure, identify the point where the drain should be placed, estimate the quantity and characteristics of the fluid, see if the pleural effusion is free or organised and prevent complications related to an incorrect manoeuvre [2].

The manoeuvre must be avoided in patients on anti-coagulant therapy until the INR is <1.5.

Before the procedure, a blood clotting profile is necessary to avoid bleeding; a non-urgent manoeuvre must be avoided in patients on anti-coagulant therapy until the INR is <1.5.

Antibiotic prophylaxis should normally not be necessary, but is recommended in the case of thoracic trauma.

The patient's signed consent to perform the procedure and a venous access are also essential.

16.4 Procedure

The procedure may be subdivided into several points.

The drain is ideally placed in the so-called 'safety triangle'.

16.4.1 Positioning of the Patient and Point of Introduction of the Drain

The patient can be positioned in lateral decubitus on the side opposite the drain insertion site with the arm above the head, or in semi-supine recumbency, always with the arm above the head (◘ Fig. 16.1). This is because the drain is ideally placed in the so-called 'safety triangle' [3]. This area is located between the middle and anterior axillary lines, in the fourth or fifth intercostal space, passing over the upper edge of the lower rib

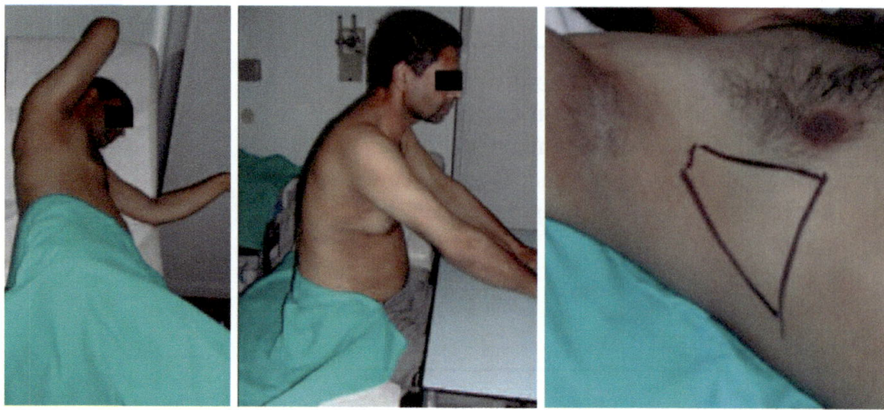

Fig. 16.1 Positioning of the patient in decubitus on the side, sitting and semi-supine

to avoid the intercostal bundle (artery, veins and nerves). The fourth intercostal space is normally at the nipple level in the male and on the inframammary line in the female. But the patient can also be positioned seated if it is decided, after TUS, that posterior access is necessary.

16.4.2 Choice of Pleural Drain

The drains are measured in French (3 French = 1 mm) and are divided into narrow drains (less than or equal to 14 French (F)) and wide drains (greater than 14 F). The narrow drains used in Italy by respiratory physicians are of two types, the Pigtail-type catheter with Seldinger technique or the Unico-type catheter with a Veress needle, while the wide drains consist of the classic Trocar (Fig. 16.2).

The use of narrow catheters has increased, favouring those positioned with the Seldinger technique.

In recent years, the use of narrow catheters has increased, favouring those positioned with the Seldinger technique. Narrow catheters have a lower risk of severe complications, are less painful for the patient and require less anaesthesia, are quicker to place and provide better patient comfort. Both pulmonologists and surgeons increasingly use these drains in patients presenting with acute symptoms secondary to pneumothorax or pleural effusion. The most frequent problem that arises with the use of small-calibre drains is the blocking of the discharge: daily washing with physiological or fibrinolytic solution is recommended. Narrow drains below 14 F are the first choice in the treatment of pneumothorax, pleural effusion and empyema. Wide drains should be used when narrower ones fail [4].

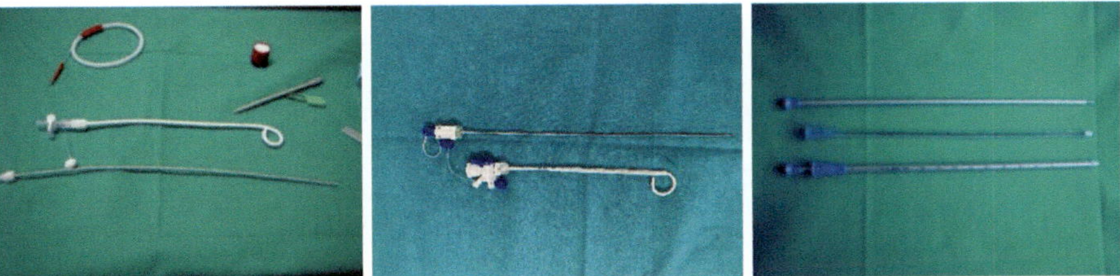

Fig. 16.2 Small-bore pig tail catheter, small-bore Unico catheter and large-bore Trocar catheter

In the case of haemothorax, for the obvious reasons linked to a high viscosity of these fluids, a wide drain is essential, of at least 28–30 F.

Narrow drains can also be left in place and managed at home in the case of relapsing malignant pleural effusion requiring frequent thoracentesis. The specifications of the narrow catheters indicate that they can be left in place for less than 2 months. If longer times are expected, it would be advisable to proceed with the placement of a tunnelled catheter.

16.4.3 Chest Drain Placement

The use of TUS is essential.

The drain is positioned in the so-called 'safety triangle'. The access point is identified through thoracic ultrasound. The use of TUS is essential, especially in complicated patients with a medical history of thoracic infections or surgery with the associated high possibility of finding adhesions or loculations. The material required for positioning a drain is indicated in Table 16.2.

During local anaesthesia, it is advisable to enter the pleural cavity with a narrow-gauge needle to check that there really is air or fluid.

- Trocar-type drain placement: for Trocar-type chest drainage, a so-called wide-bore chest tube is used. The most used gauge is 20 or 24 F. This is an 'armed' drain, made rigid by a mandrel positioned inside it in order to facilitate penetration of the chest wall and positioning within the pleural cavity. The procedure manoeuvre must be performed in sterility to avoid infections. First of all, local anaesthesia is practised (20 mL of 2% xylocaine, first on the surface, then subcutaneously) which can be associated with analgesics (NSAIDs, tramadol, morphine) and sedatives (midazolam) in case of failure to control painful symptoms. It is emphasised that, during local anaesthesia, it is advisable to enter the pleural cavity with a narrow-gauge needle to check that there really is air or fluid. A cutaneous and subcutaneous incision is then made longitudinally along the course of the

Table 16.2 Material needed to place a thoracic drain

1. Sterile gloves and sterile gowns
2. Antiseptic solution
3. Sterile sheets to delimit the disinfected skin area
4. Sterile gauze
5. Syringes and needles (21–25 gauge)
6. Xylocaine 2%
7. Scalpel
8. Suture thread
9. Instruments for minor surgery including 'blunt tip' scissors
10. Drains of various sizes
11. Connection pipes, biconical valves and drainage system

ribs, of the size of the drain that will be introduced, being careful not to sink the scalpel blade too deep so as to avoid vascular injury. Immediately after, a controlled dissection through the intercostal muscles is made using blunt-tipped scissors or a Kelly clamp, creating a track extending over the top and into the intercostal space and opening up the pleural surface. At this point, the Trocar is introduced, which will be directed towards the apex of the lung in the case of pneumothorax or towards the base in the case of pleural effusion. The drain will be connected to an aspiration system. Finally, it will be necessary to fix the drainage tube to the chest wall, to avoid accidental leakage, by applying a linear suture perpendicular to the incision line. The placement of the drain should then be checked with a chest X-ray in the two views.

The dilator should not be inserted further than 1 cm.

- Small-bore drain placement with Seldinger's technique: Another type of drainage is the small-bore 'pig-tail' 14 F catheter introduced with the Seldinger technique [5]. After locating the insertion position, local anaesthetic (lidocaine 2%) should be infiltrated in the cutaneous and subcutaneous layers. During this procedure, an attempt should be made to aspirate the pleural contents with a narrow-gauge needle. If this is not possible, chest drain insertion should not continue. Once fluid or air is found, a small incision is made with a scalpel blade. The needle (supplied with the Seldinger kit) is then inserted into the intercostal space to penetrate the pleural space. Air or pleural fluid should be aspirated via the needle. The syringe is removed and the guide wire is passed through the needle; there should be no resistance and the wire should pass freely. The needle is then removed and the guide wire left in. The dilator is passed over the guide wire into the thorax. The dilator should not be inserted further than 1 cm beyond the depth from the skin to the pleural space. The dilator is then removed, ensuring that the wire is not pulled out of, or pushed further into, the thorax. The drain is inserted by sliding it over the guide wire, to approximately 12–16 cm. The guide wire and inner tube are then removed from the drain.

16.4.4 Indwelling Pleural Catheters (IPCs)

The expected benefit is the management of the patient at home.

Indwelling pleural catheters are used with increasing frequency in the treatment of malignant pleural effusion [6]. The catheter is tunnelled under the skin to the pleural space. The main function of the IPC is that it can remain in place for a much longer period of time compared to normal drainage. The expected benefit is the management of the patient at home, thus avoiding repeated thoracentesis and entailing the reduction of hospitalisation times. Their use can also be extended to chronic benign effusions such as hepatic hydrothorax and inflammatory pleuritis.

IPCs are placed under local anaesthesia and are then managed at home by trained caregivers, who will have to remove the fluid using special vacuum bottles.

There are some negative aspects: first of all the high costs, then the risk of pleural cavity infections, malfunctioning, the formation of a loculated pleural collection and the risk of metastasis along the path of the catheter.

16.5 Drainage Systems

The chest drain should be connected to a drainage system that incorporates a valve mechanism to prevent air or fluid from entering the pleural cavity..

- *Heimlich valve*. The simplest system is that of the Heimlich valve (◘ Fig. 16.3). It consists of a cylinder of plastic material measuring a few centimetres in length, with an opening on each of the two bases. Inside the cylinder, there is a collapsible rubber tube connected to one of the openings. This opening must be connected to the drain, and the other opening must be left open. The use of the Heimlich valve, however, is limited to pneumothorax, as the presence

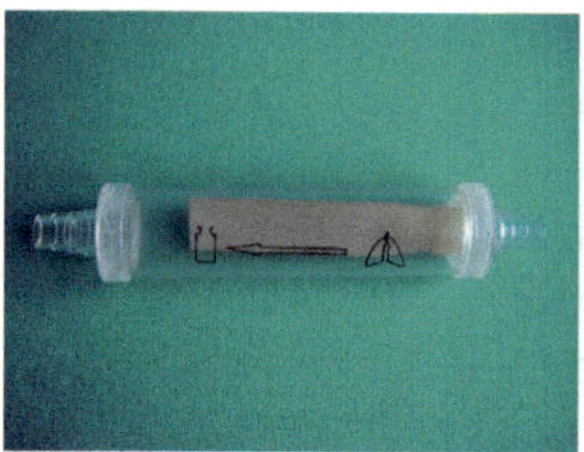
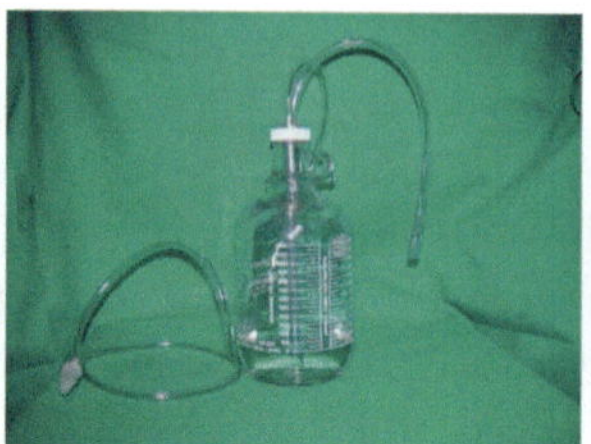
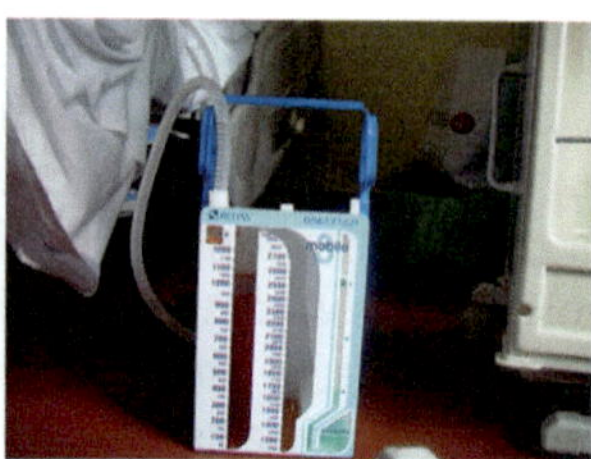

Fig. 16.3 Heimlich valve, Bulau-type water valve, Redax-type collection system

The most commonly used drainage system is the Bulau bottle-type water valve

of fluid material, disturbing the clearance of the valves, can affect their functioning.

- *Bulau valve*. The most commonly used drainage system is the Bulau bottle-type water valve (Fig. 16.3). The system consists of a bottle equipped with a screw cap through which two tubes are inserted: the longer tube reaches the bottom of the bottle, and the short tube ends just under the cap. The Bulau valve must contain physiological solution or sterile water so that the long tube is immersed in it for at least 2 cm. The long tube connects to the patient drain. The shorter tube, not immersed in the fluid, must allow the air to escape and must be left open or connected to the aspiration system. The increase in intrapleural pressure in the expiratory phase enables the escape of air or fluid from the pleural cavity. In the event of a pleural effusion, fluid accumulates in the bottle. In the case of pneumothorax, the air, after being 'bubbled' through the sterile water that acts as a valve and which is contained in the Bulau valve, comes out through the short tube (the open one).
- *Redax*. When large quantities of fluid come out of the pleural cavity, it is advisable to use a two-bottle system, one bottle serving to collect the fluid while the other serves as a water valve. A single closed system called Redax (Fig. 16.3) can also be used, which combines both the water valve and the container for collecting the fluid in the same box.
- *Pleur Evac*. This is a very handy single-use system that can function as a three-bottle system. The first column on the right corresponds to the collection bottle, the second column to the water valve, and the third column to the pressure control bottle. It is a system used above all by surgeons in post-operative care.

16.6 Negative Pressure Aspiration

Negative pressure aspiration at levels of 10 to 20 cm H_2O can be applied to the drainage system. The application of negative pressure is necessary above all in two situations: in the case of pneumothorax with substantial leaks or after pleurodesis. After pleurodesis with talc, an aspiration with negative pressure of at least 10 to 20 cm H_2O must be applied. The patient has to stay in bed connected to the aspirator continuously for the first 24 h, crucial for the success of the pleurodesis [7].

16.7 Removal of Drain

The drain should be removed when drained fluid is less than 200 mL/day, at resolution of pneumothorax, or if drainage fails. After the drain has been removed, the cutaneous passage is closed with stitches or Steri Strips and then medicated with gauze.

The drain should be removed when drained fluid is less than 200 mL/day.

16.8 Complications

Complications include pain, bleeding, superficial site infection, deep infection of the pleural cavity (empyema), accidental removal of the tube, clogging of the drain, pulmonary re-expansion oedema, placement in the incorrect anatomic position with secondary trauma of abdominal organs such as the spleen or liver, and trauma of the diaphragm or of intrathoracic organs such as the aorta or heart. With the use of a small-bore Seldinger drain, the incidence of placement in the incorrect anatomic position and organ injury will hopefully be reduced. On the other hand, given the persistence of complications in the various cases described above and the widespread availability of ultrasound equipment, it is recommended that you always use a US scan to place a thoracic drain, reducing the incidence of complications [8].

References

1. Porcel JM. Chest tube drainage of the pleural space: a concise review for pulmonologists. Tuberc Respir Dis (Seoul). 2018;81(2):106–15. https://doi.org/10.4046/trd.2017.0107. Epub 2018 Jan 24. PMID: 29372629; PMCID: PMC5874139.

2. Toma TP, Trigiani M, Zanforlin A, Inchingolo R, Zanobetti M, Sammicheli L, Conte EG, Buggio G, Villari L, Corbetta L, Marchetti G. Competence in thoracic ultrasound. Panminerva Med. 2019;61(3):344–66. https://doi.org/10.23736/S0031-0808.18.03577-2. Epub 2018 Nov 27. PMID: 30486618.
3. Laws D, Neville E, Duffy J, Pleural Diseases Group, Standards of Care Committee, British Thoracic Society. BTS guidelines for the insertion of a chest drain. Thorax. 2003;58(Suppl. 2):ii53–9. https://doi.org/10.1136/thorax.58.suppl_2.ii53. PMID: 12728150; PMCID: PMC1766017.
4. Carlucci P, Trigiani M, Mori PA, Mondoni M, Pinelli V, Casalini AG, Conte EG, Buggio G, Villari L, Marchetti G. Competence in pleural procedures. Panminerva Med. 2019;61(3):326–43. https://doi.org/10.23736/S0031-0808.18.03564-4. Epub 2018 Oct 31. PMID: 30394712.
5. Mori PA, Casalini AG, Miglio V. Il drenaggio toracico. In: Casalini AG, editor. Pneumologia Interventistica. Milan: Springer; 2007. p. 555–66.
6. Bertolaccini L, Viti A, Paiano S, Pomari C, Assante LR, Terzi A. Indwelling pleural catheters: a clinical option in trapped lung. Thorac Surg Clin. 2017;27(1):47–55. https://doi.org/10.1016/j.thorsurg.2016.08.008. PMID: 27865327.
7. Mori PA, Casalini AG. Therapeutic medical thoracoscopy. Monaldi Arch Chest Dis. 2011;75(1):89–94. PMID: 21627003.
8. Santos C, Gupta S, Baraket M, Collett PJ, Xuan W, Williamson JP. Outcomes of an initiative to improve inpatient safety of small bore thoracostomy tube insertion. Intern Med J. 2019;49(5):644–9. https://doi.org/10.1111/imj.14110. PMID: 30230151; PMCID: PMC6851751.

Clinical Case of Pleural Effusion with an Interesting Ultrasound Picture

G. P. Marchetti

Contents

A. G. Casalini (ed.), *Practical Manual of Pleural Pathology*,
https://doi.org/10.1007/978-3-031-20312-1_17

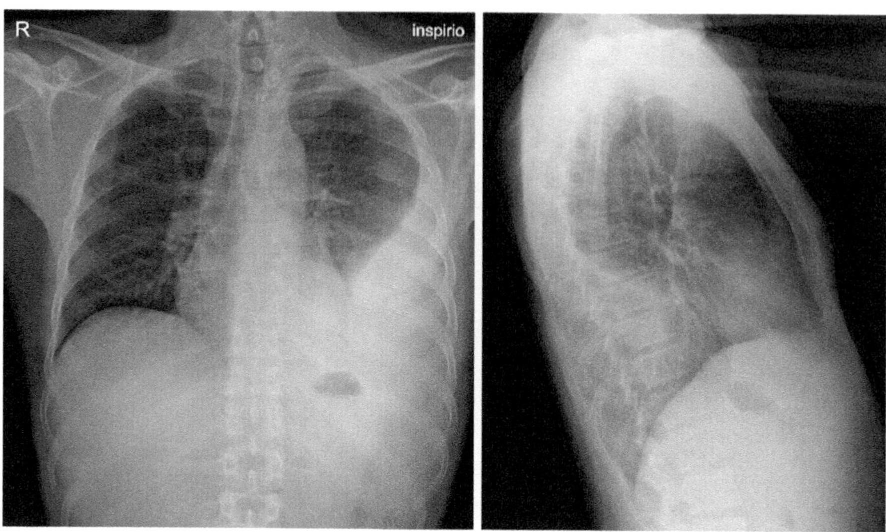

■ **Fig. 17.1** Chest X-ray at admission to emergency department

We here present the clinical case of a 50-year-old Indian man, an agricultural labourer and a non-smoker, with a negative past medical history. For about 1 week, the patient had had a dry cough, fever (max 38 °C) and pain in the left chest [1]. He therefore went to the Emergency Department of our hospital, where a chest X-ray was taken, which showed the presence of left, non-free flowing, loculated, posterior pleural effusion (■ Fig. 17.1). He was admitted to Pneumology.

There was nothing significant in blood laboratory tests; the C-reactive protein was 61 mg/L.

With the patient in a sitting position, pulmonary ultrasound was performed, showing modest anechoic and fibrinous, posterior, left pleural effusion visible in two intercostal spaces. There was a 1-mm thickening of the parietal pleura in the postero-inferior quadrants and the presence in the parasternal area of the left sub-clavicular region of an enlarged internal mammary lymph node with a transverse diameter greater than 1.1 cm [2] (■ Fig. 17.2).

An exploratory thoracentesis was thus performed, with the aspiration of 50 mL of yellowish pleural fluid, on which a cytological examination was performed with the differential cell count: lymphocytes were 95%. In the strong suspicion of tuberculous pleurisy, medical thoracoscopy was performed under local anaesthesia with the introduction of an ultrasound-guided Trocar in the sixth intercostal space on the posterior axillary line [3]. Even in the presence of a cytological result strongly indicative of tuberculosis, we consider it essential to immediately perform a diagnostic medical thoracoscopy, a

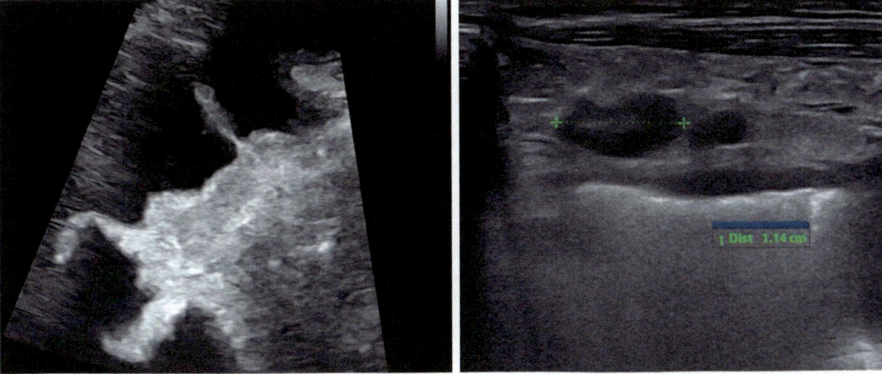

■ **Fig. 17.2** Thoracic ultrasound: left, fibrinous effusion; right, internal mammary lymph node enlarged in left parasternal region

simple procedure in the hands of an expert pulmonologist that yields histological and microbiological material (on tissue and fibrin) which, if positive for *M. tuberculosis*, allows for all microbiological examinations and for cultures and possible drug resistance test [4]. The advantages of early thoracoscopy are innumerable: the examination becomes simple and fast, the diagnosis becomes absolutely certain, and the cleaning of the pleural cavity reduces the possibility of a negative pleural outcome such as pleural thickening.

After aspiration of 1000 cm^3 of cloudy pleural fluid, the pleural cavity was explored, with the finding of some fresh, soft, fluctuating adhesions of whitish and avascular fibrin. We therefore proceeded to a mechanical lavage with saline solution and removal of the membranes for subsequent microbiological examination. The parietal and diaphragmatic pleurae were ubiquitously hyperaemic, friable and covered with dense, low-relief, salmon-coloured granulations (■ Fig. 17.3). The presence of millimetre-sized nodules in all quadrants was clearly visible with the optic light; this classic "strawberry" appearance already heavily pointed towards tuberculosis. Multiple biopsies were performed in several places, taking material for both microbiological and histological examination. The manoeuvre was concluded with the placement of a 20-French chest drain. The patient had no complications at the end of the procedure.

The CT scan performed after the thoracoscopy showed, in addition to a clear reduction in the pleural effusion, a very modest irregular thickening at the left base and a homogeneous, reactive, oval 12 mm lymph node of the left internal mammary chain (■ Fig. 17.4); there were no significant parenchymal alterations, no atelectasis from compression and a complete absence of cavity lesions.

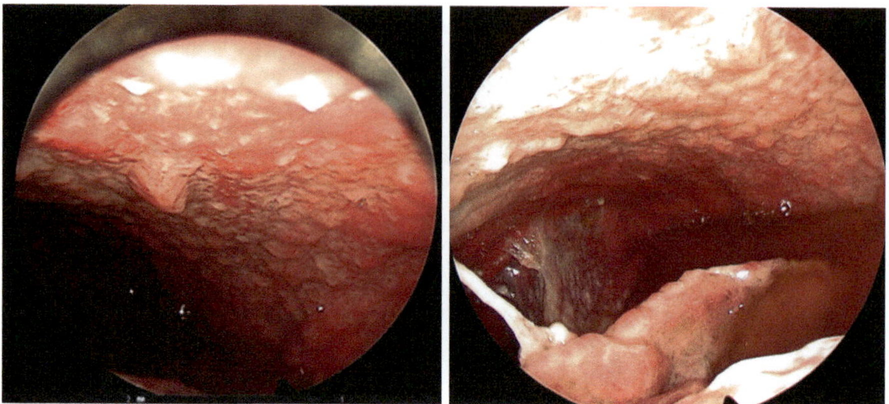

Fig. 17.3 Endoscopic picture at medical thoracoscopy

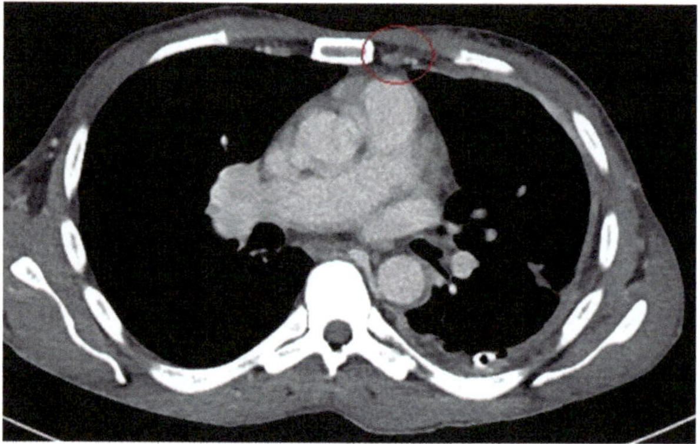

Fig. 17.4 Chest CT

The microbiological examination of the pleural fluid was negative.

The histological examination showed the presence of numerous granulomas with focal necrosis, fibrin and tissue negative for *M. tuberculosis* both direct and cultured. This datum, too—granulomas in the absence of microbiological confirmation—enhances the importance of the pleural biopsy, which should always be performed.

The patient then began anti-tuberculous therapy according to protocol, with four drugs (Rifampicin, Isoniazid, Ethambutol and Pyrazinamide).

On the third day, the thoracic drain was removed, and the patient was discharged in good clinical condition. Complete blood count and liver function tests 10 days after discharge were recommended.

Two-monthly outpatient check-ups were scheduled.

Conclusive Comments

The presence of a suspected infectious pleurisy, associated with fever and with a fibrinous effusion on ultrasound examination, points to a possible tuberculous pleurisy if non-specific phlogosis indices are negative (no leukocytosis and moderately elevated CRP), in contrast to the classic bacterial-infectious pleurisy, where the leukocyte values are typically high and the CRP values are much higher.

If the pleural fluid has lymphocytosis >50%, there is a high possibility of tuberculous pleurisy.

The presence of fibrinous, light and fluctuating loculations, as well as of at least one lymph node of the internal mammary chain with a major axis greater than 0.5 cm associated with a pleural lymphocytosis >50%, has a high positive predictive value for tuberculous pleurisy.

Pulmonologists who manage patients with pleural effusion and suspected TB must be able to identify the presence of a pathological internal mammary lymph node on ultrasound even in the absence of a CT scan.

Medical thoracoscopy is the gold-standard exam that enables the histological and microbiological analysis of the pleuro-pulmonary tissue and fibrin, and should always be performed in the presence of pleural lymphocytosis and pathological breast lymph node [4].

The presence of pleural granulomas and clinical compatibility, even without direct and cultural isolation of M. tuberculosis, warrants the initiation of anti-mycobacterial therapy with four drugs.

References

1. Jane A. Tuberculous pleural effusion. Respirology. 2019;24:962. https://doi.org/10.1111/resp.13673.
2. Shaw JA, Diacon AH, Koegelenberg CFN. Tuberculous pleural effusion. Respirology. 2019;24(10):962–71. https://doi.org/10.1111/resp.13673. Epub 2019 Aug 16. PMID: 31418985.
3. Messineo L, Quadri F, Valsecchi A, Lonni S, Palmiotti A, Marchetti G. Internal mammary lymph node visualization as a sentinel sonographic sign of tuberculous pleurisy. Ultraschall Med. 2019;40(4):488–94. https://doi.org/10.1055/a-0879-1758. English. Epub 2019 Jun 25. PMID: 31238381.
4. Casalini AG, et al. Pleural tuberculosis: medical thoracoscopy greatly increases the diagnostic accuracy. ERJ Open Res Act. 2018;4(1):00046–2017. https://doi.org/10.1183/23120541.00046-2017.

Transthoracic Ultrasound in Pleural Diseases

G. P. Marchetti

Contents

A. G. Casalini (ed.), *Practical Manual of Pleural Pathology*,
https://doi.org/10.1007/978-3-031-20312-1_18

18.1 Introduction

The pleura was the first thoracic structure to be studied with ultrasound.

The simplest and most immediate field of application of transthoracic ultrasound is the study of the pleura. Pulmonologists were slow to discover this precious resource, which had already aided 'difficult' thoracentesis since the 1970s, the first ever successfully performed by cardiologists [1]. In recent years, the use of pleural ultrasound has become increasingly routine due to its dynamism and simplicity [2], low cost and freedom from ionising radiation; it is repeatable, now compatible with light and portable instruments, and easy to handle and to perform [3]. It has been shown to provide diagnostic information in a short time and to assist both doctor and nurse during invasive manoeuvres, both in the endoscopic room and at the patient's bedside. It has become an irreplaceable resource before and during thoracoscopy [4] and has been able to identify with certainty and speed some complications of Interventional Pulmonology such as pneumothorax or haemothorax (■ Table 18.1).

■ **Table 18.1** Advantages in pleural ultrasound

Ultrasound in pleural diseases: why?
• Easy learning
• No radiation
• Autonomy
• Real time
• Fast
• Very useful in babies and children
• Possible in pregnant women
• Takes advantage of decubitus and gravity
• 70% of pleural surface visible
• Fundamental in the follow-up
• Fundamental in invasive manoeuvres
• Fundamental in the evaluation of infectious effusions

18.2 Technique

The difference of acoustic impedance between the thoracic wall and the air present inside the lung makes the pleural surface easily identifiable; however, this acoustic barrier unfortunately makes it impossible, in the absence of pathology, to see the organ in-depth [5].

The two probes that best allow us to study lung diseases are:

- the convex probe, at low frequency (3.5 MHz), which allows for greater depth, reaching a depth of up to 15 cm, enabling a panoramic view of the effusion. Alternatively, the 2.5 MHz cardiac sector probe can be used. These types of probe are indispensable in the evaluation of effusion, as a guide to interventional procedures and in the study of diaphragmatic motility.
- the linear probe, at high frequency (7–15 MHz), which provides an image with a higher resolution but reaches a depth of only a few cm. This probe is very useful for a more in-depth study of the pleural surfaces and their sliding, in pneumothorax in search of the lung point (PTX), in identifying plaques and pleural thickening, and in the search for minimal pleural effusions in the costophrenic sinuses.

The convex probe for effusion and its characteristics, the linear one for thoracic wall and pneumothorax

The only limitations to ultrasound exploration are the presence of subcutaneous emphysema and the inability to explore some thoracic regions such as the retro-scapular, apical and supra-diaphragmatic regions. It is estimated that 70% of the pleural surface can be explored by ultrasound.

70% of the pleural surface can be studied with ultrasound.

Regarding the way the examination is performed, patients are preferably studied in a sitting position, which facilitates the search for a pleural effusion due to gravity, and in the supine one to explore the sub-clavicular regions in search of pneumothorax [6].

In healthy subjects, the parietal and visceral serosa together form an interface with a thickness of several hundreds of microns known as the pleural line, and we must start from this to begin our evaluation and then interpret the disease [7].

The pleural line is the main target to look for before any other.

The pleural line is a horizontal and luminous line a few centimetres from the skin, hyperechoic and brilliant, that normally moves synchronously with the breath that in longitudinal scan is seen between the ribs, while in the oblique one it is totally visible. This movement is called 'sliding' and is maximum at the base and more contained at the apex; its absence is almost always a sign of pneumothorax. It may also be absent in previous pleurodesis, pneumo/lobectomies and fibrothorax.

Ultrasound, the only diagnostic test, studies the pleura in motion.

The ventilated pulmonary base that moves during the acts of breath covering the abdominal organs, on the other hand, constitutes the 'curtain sign' whose width on the right is clearly visible and measurable. The pleural line can move synchronously with the heartbeat, especially to the left, and this movement is more accentuated if the lung is consolidated [8].

All signs of normality and pathology depart from the pleural line, the true protagonist of thoracic ultrasound. In the normal lung, thin horizontal artefactual lines (A lines) repeat evenly and parallel below the pleural surface, while B lines are vertical hyperechoic reflections extending from the pleural line to the edge of the screen image. They move in synchrony with sliding and when present they attenuate until the A lines are cancelled. The presence of the B lines is synonymous with 'interstitial syndrome' caused by a decrease in air content and an increase in lung density, as occurs in the presence of pneumonia, pulmonary oedema, fibrosis, ARDS, neoplastic carcinosis and alveolar haemorrhages [9].

18.3 Pleural Effusion

Chest ultrasound is considered the 'gold standard' for the study of pleural effusion.

Chest ultrasound is considered the 'gold standard' for the study of pleural effusion (◘ Fig. 18.1). The ultrasound examination guides the diagnostic and therapeutic strategy. In fact, in at least half of pleural effusions, there is a 'change' in the diagnostic and therapeutic management after the patient has undergone ultrasound. The pleural fluid is easily identifiable due to the presence of different degrees of echogenicity compared to other body tissues. Ultrasound is not only useful for its easy identification but is an essential tool for a more in-depth analysis of the effusion. It enables its exact location and its arrangement within the chest, as well as freedom of movement with the decubitus, allows for a very reliable estimate of the entity and evaluates the specific echogenic characteristics [10].

The scan, preferably oblique, must start from the base, always identifying as a reference the acoustic windows of the liver on the right and the spleen on the left. Free effusion accumulates by gravity and moves along with the decubitus; it is visible first in the costophrenic angle and as it increases it fills the cavity by leaning on the lower lobe and progressively squeezing it towards the hilum. The parenchyma gradually loses its air content and is visible as a solid, floating structure within the fluid (the 'jellyfish sign'). These ultrasound signs indicate that this lung will most likely undergo re-expansion after thoracentesis. If, on the other hand, the lung is 'trapped',

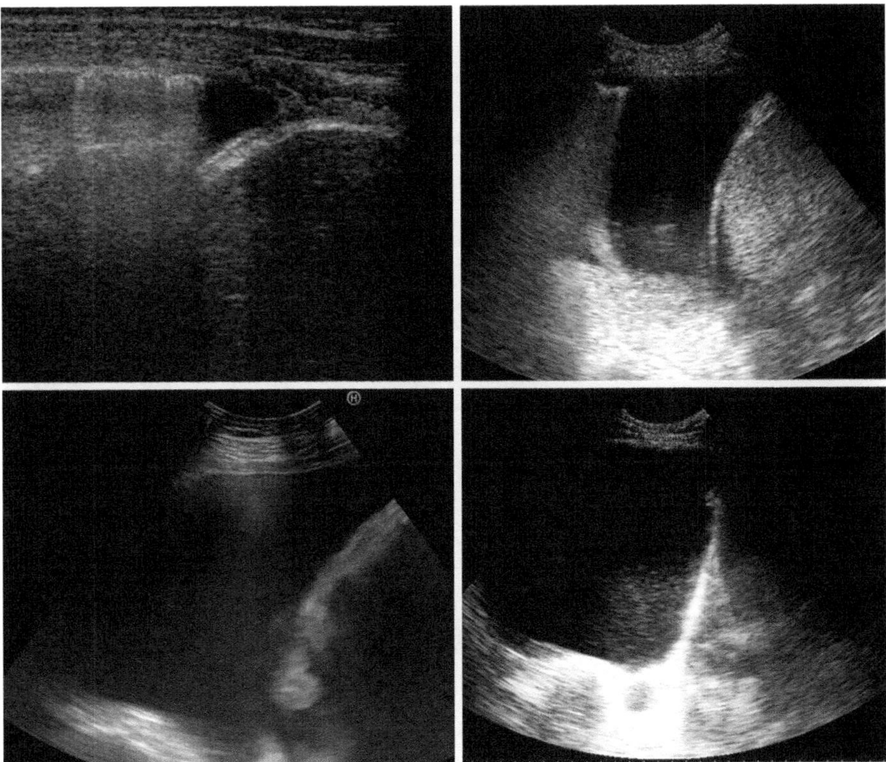

Fig. 18.1 Free pleural effusions

it assumes a rigid shape, not very mobile, with hyperechoic contours, and in all probability will not re-expand during the evacuation manoeuvre [11].

Dyspnoea can easily be distinguished as to cardiogenic or pulmonary origin.

It is difficult to quantify exactly the volume of an effusion; there are various formulas but nevertheless they are seldom applied. The complex geometry of the chest and the variable constitution of the patients are obstacles to the exact estimation of the amount of fluid. An approximate measurement is expressed as 'light' if visible in only one intercostal space, 'moderate' if it occupies two intercostal spaces and 'massive' if it is seen in three or more spaces [12]. Ultrasound allows us to identify very small amounts of fluid (5 mL), whereas the chest X-ray is able to detect the effusion when at least 150 mL or more are present. A linear probe, by studying the costo-phrenic sinus, can also look for the presence of pleural adhesions or irregularities, thus increasing the probability that we are faced with a neoplastic form, while the presence of fibrin almost always identifies the infectious and/or inflammatory effusions (Fig. 18.2). It is always useful to place the probe also in the contralateral hemithorax, as the bilateral nature of the fluid

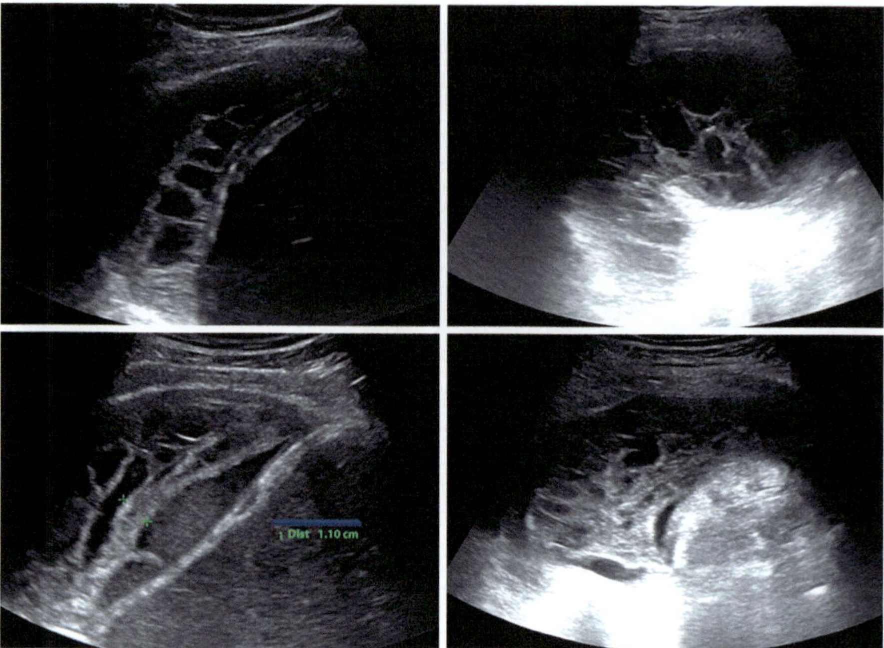

Fig. 18.2 Parapneumonic effusion

has a great diagnostic value. In the presence of bilateral effusion, it is also necessary to evaluate the diameter of the inferior vena cava and its collapsibility with the acts of breathing, in order to rule out heart failure.

The fluid can be anechoic (and this does not mean transudate) or may contain within it more or less rigid membranes that loculate it, which can be free or fixed, thick or thin, single or multiple; pulmonary ultrasound is much more sensitive than CT for their identification. In the presence of empyema (Fig. 18.3), on the other hand, the echogenicity is very high, similar to that of the liver, sometimes granular and irregular, and there may be air inside it.

In infectious effusion, ultrasound is more sensitive than CT to decide the treatment.

The loculations are typical of acute and bacterial infectious effusion (Fig. 18.2), and the ultrasound dictates the behaviour to be followed: when to drain and how, which drain to use, the best position, whether to use fibrinolytics, when to decide to remove it. Septations, albeit rarely, can also occur in long-standing exudations, but can also be found in neoplastic pleural cavities, mesothelioma and especially lung neoplasms.

Tuberculous pleurisy, on the other hand, is ultrasonographically different. There is less fibrin, sometimes a millimetre of irregular parietal thickening is visible, and in almost all cases the presence of an enlarged internal mammary chain lymph node is detectable (Fig. 18.4).

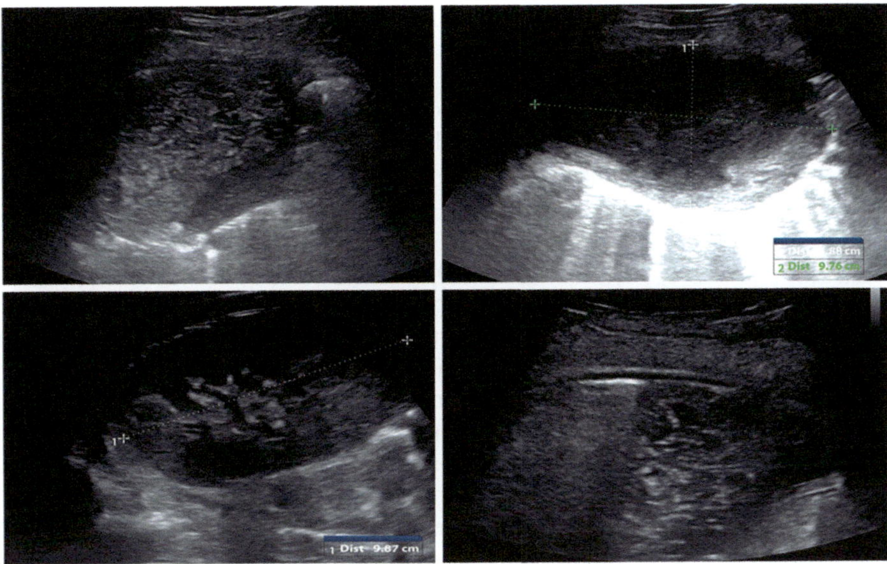

Fig. 18.3 Empyema

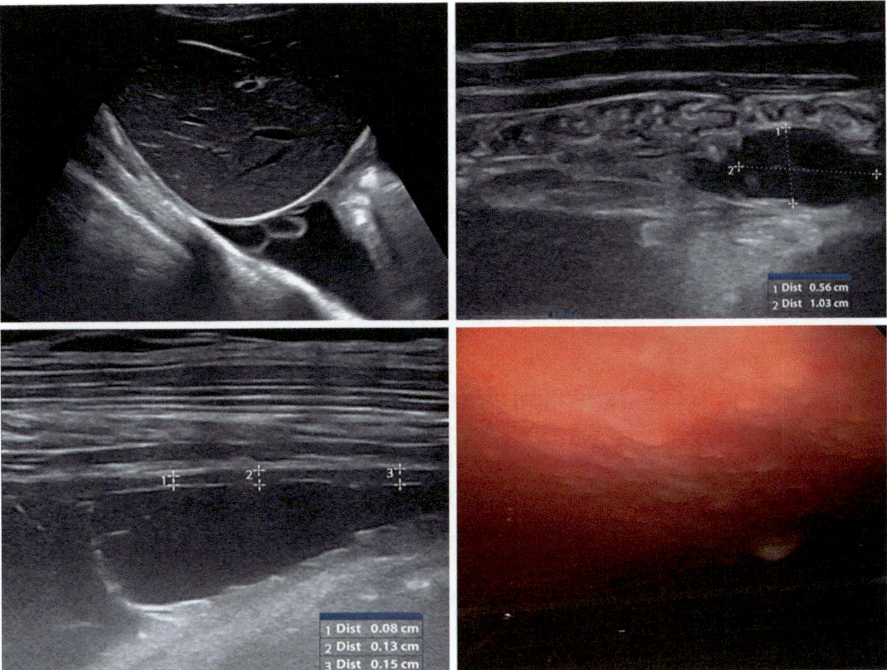

Fig. 18.4 Pleural tuberculosis

The presence of fluid makes visible the diaphragm and lung parenchyma, which can be the site of collateral anomalies such as nodules, infiltrations or parenchymal abscesses. The absence of air-bronchograms inside the collapsed lung and its rigidity may lead to the suspicion of atelectasis or 'trapped lung' [13].

18.4 Pneumothorax

Pneumothorax is easily identifiable, especially in urgency.

Ultrasound diagnosis of pneumothorax (PNX), with very high sensitivity and specificity, must be included among the most recent and most clinically useful achievements. The possibility of making a safe and quick diagnosis at the patient's bedside has a very high value in this disease. Although CT remains the gold standard, ultrasound has become a safe and reliable procedure, overtaking traditional radiology [14].

The signs are many and pathognomonic, reliable and safe: first of all, the absence of sliding and the disappearance of B-lines; the increase in horizontal artefacts; where possible, the identification of the 'lung point' (that is, the exact point where the parenchyma detaches from the wall); the disappearance of the lung-pulse [15]. Since the free air collects in the upper spaces, the PNX should be sought with the linear probe anteriorly in the sub-clavicular area with the patient in the supine position. The pleural spaces should be explored longitudinally from the sternum to the mid-clavicular line and from the clavicle to the anterior diaphragm. This ultrasound picture can be part of a differential diagnosis with some conditions of reduced lung compliance where sliding is reduced, such as atelectasis or a congenital or acquired symphysis.

18.5 Thickening and Neoplasia

Another anomaly that can be easily identified with ultrasound is the thickening of the serosa. It appears as an echo-free stripe that moves the pleural line deeply. It is essential to evaluate the edges and infiltration towards the thoracic wall but also in the parenchyma; the irregularity and depth raise the suspicion of neoplasia, mainly mesothelioma. However, the edges are smooth and respect the sliding in the benign forms, as in asbestos hyaline plaques. In fact, pleural hyaline plaques usually appear as hypo-anechoic, elliptical and smooth lesions, not modified by the decubitus, the diaphragmatic ones being the most difficult to identify. Inside them, there may be calcifications that occur with the typical posterior acoustic shadowing [16].

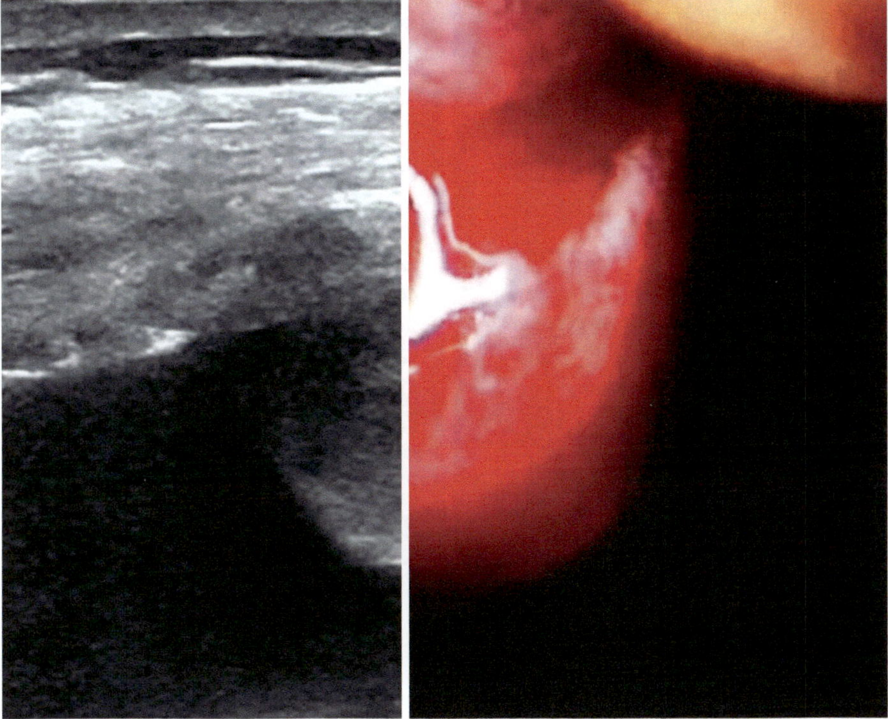

Fig. 18.5 Metastatic nodule

Another extensive field in which ultrasound diagnosis has acquired increasing importance is that of pleuro-pulmonary neoplasms, primary and secondary, whether associated with pleural effusion or not (Fig. 18.5).

A thorough scan can allow for the precise definition of the localisation of the tumour (extrapleural, pleural or parenchymal), local infiltration, the extent of the mass and its nature (solid, cystic or complex) (Fig. 18.6).

Extrapleural tumours move the pleural line deeply by deviating its underlying straight profile and are often associated with destruction of the ribs or muscle infiltration. If, on the other hand, the lesions are in the cavity, it is necessary to distinguish the pleural ones that do not move with sliding but respect it from the peripheral pulmonary ones that instead tend to move with the breath. On the other hand, the identification of central tumours is impossible due to the interposition of an aerated lung between the lesion and the probe. The invasion of the wall can be evaluated more accurately with ultrasound than with CT [17].

Malignant mesothelioma arises in the pleural cavity and ultrasound can detect it at an early stage (Fig. 18.7).

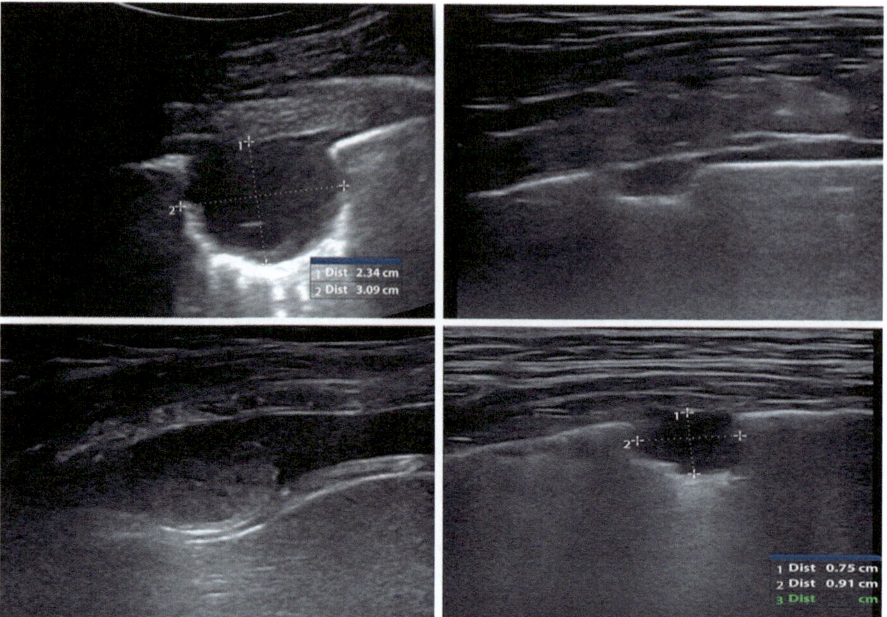

Fig. 18.6 Intrathoracic metastasis

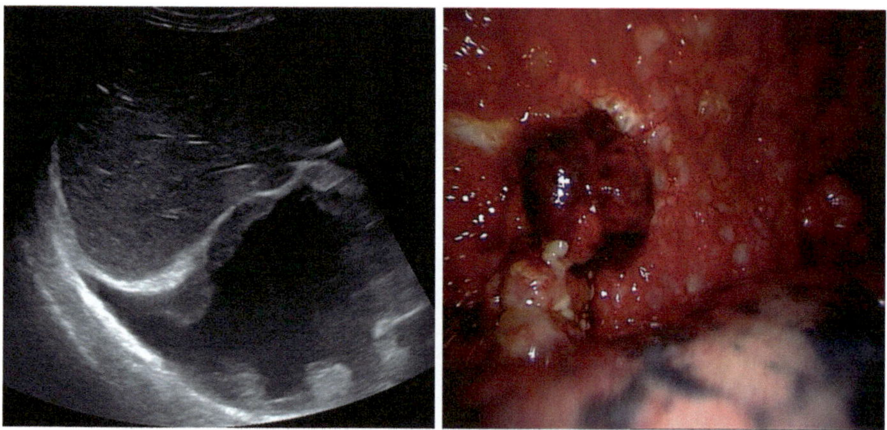

Fig. 18.7 Malignant mesothelioma

Attention should always be paid to the costo-phrenic sinus, the real thermometer of the pleural cavity. It should be studied in all positions: if there is fluid, it acts as a contrast for the possible presence of a suspicious thickening or even better for neoplastic nodulation, generally with a large implant base. We

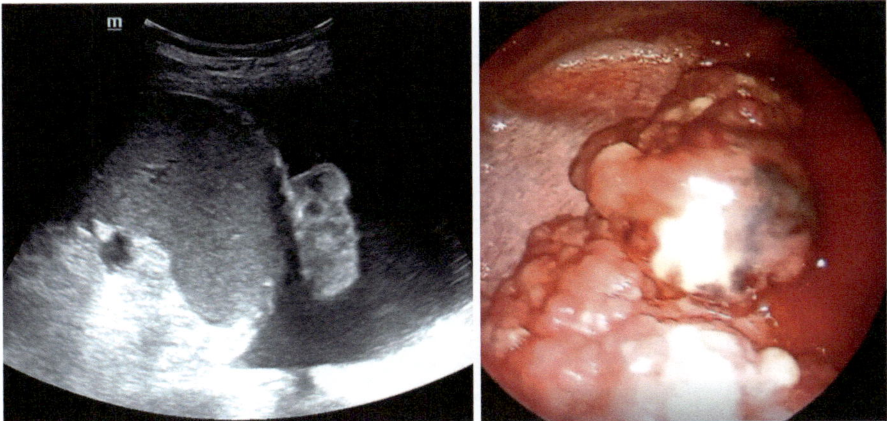

Fig. 18.8 Invasion of the diaphragm by mesothelioma

must also remember that a thickening should be placed in a differential diagnosis with the sub-pleural fat, always present above all anteriorly, and also with the physiological diaphragmatic pillars, which, however, can be modified in shape and size with the respiratory cycle. In mesothelioma, pleural effusion is almost always unilateral and associated with a history of asbestos exposure; it almost always presents as a hypo-anechoic thickening with irregular edges, which can range from a few millimetres to several centimetres, sometimes visible as a single mass, other times already boundless in the abdomen and infiltrating the thoracic wall. Its growth is variable and ultrasound is able to evaluate its evolution. The diaphragm is another excellent ultrasound window in the suspicion of mesothelioma (Fig. 18.8): It can be studied both obliquely near the sliding and subcostally. Its irregularity and thickening (greater than 5 mm) warrant a further diagnostic step, especially if in the presence of fluid (Fig. 18.9).

The concomitant search for lamellar pleural plaques in the most usual sites, such as the retromammary site, is important. The associated fluid is usually corpuscular and moderately echogenic but can be completely anechoic, with the rare but possible concomitant presence of abundant fibrin which can simulate an infectious genesis. Mesothelioma frequently shows laminar progression, which differentiates it from pleural metastases. Locally advanced cancer can invade the chest wall as well as the sites of previous drains or needle or trocar entries and ultrasound can precisely study the anatomy [18].

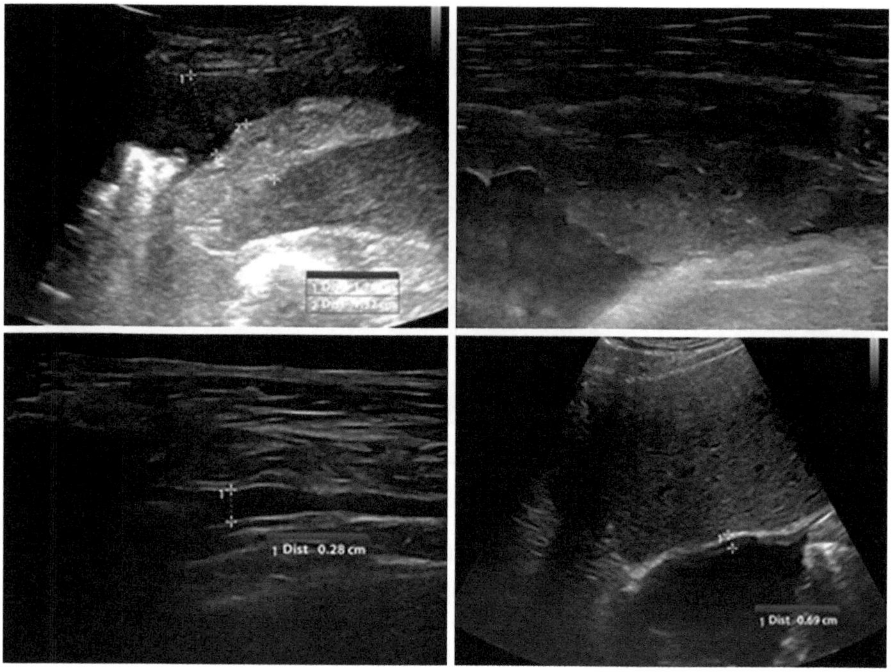

■ **Fig. 18.9** Thickening of diaphragm by mesothelioma

18.6 Interventional Ultrasound

Its role in interventional pulmonology is irreplaceable.

Interventional ultrasound (US) has proved to be fundamental as a safe and reliable guide in 'real-time' interventional manoeuvres, from simple thoracentesis to the correct positioning of a drain. In addition, thoracic ultrasound has become an indispensable tool for planning medical thoracoscopy in difficult cases, when for example there is pleural irregularity and the strong suspicion of neoplasm without the presence of fluid (■ Fig. 18.10).

With the ultrasound support, the classic 'safety triangle' has been re-sized; even areas such as the paravertebral, anterior and upper axillary ones can be safely and effectively used for access [19].

Thoracentesis, a routine and simple act, should always be performed with ultrasound guidance, studying the area chosen first with the convex probe to delimit the limits of the effusion and its relationships with the nearby parenchyma, and then with the linear probe with the Doppler probe to delineate the vascularisation of the wall in the area chosen for the puncture. It is preferable to insert the needle freehand and immediately afterwards follow the outflow of the fluid by identifying the tip of the needle throughout the manoeuvre. It is a good idea to

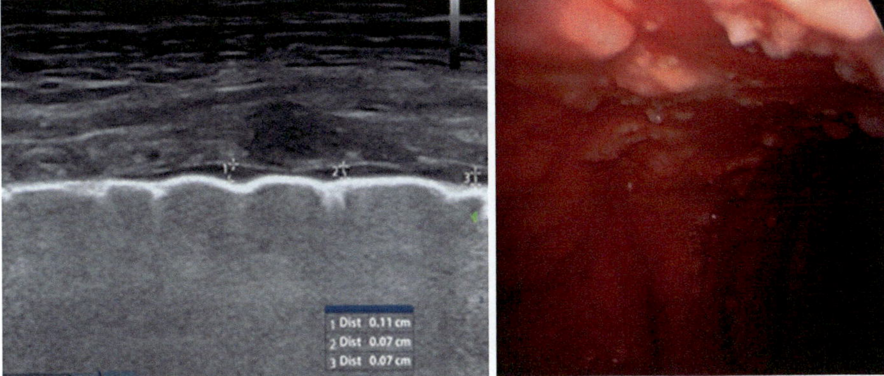

Fig. 18.10 Small nodules in ovarian pleural metastasis

introduce the needle halfway between the lower and upper limits of the effusion so that the diaphragm rising during the manoeuvre does not touch the needle. Ultrasound-guided thoracentesis has not eliminated complications such as pneumothorax or haemothorax, although it has greatly reduced them, making the procedure extremely safe.

Equal effectiveness is achieved in the positioning of the echo-guided drain, both small and large calibre. 'Difficult' areas such as the posterior paravertebral site, and those of complicated and rigid loculated effusions, are reachable in echo-guiding, as are the anterior areas. Visualisation of the drain is relatively simple although not always possible [20].

Ultrasound can also guide biopsies of chest wall lesions (Fig. 18.11), pleural thickening and nodules, but also of peripheral lung lesions that are in direct contact with the visceral pleura.

Reliability is similar to that performed with a CT guide but with enormous time savings and without exposing the patient and operator to ionising radiation. There are fixed guides to be applied to the probe that direct the needle by creating a track on the screen but sometimes make the system more rigid. The 'free hand' technique with the lateral needle and its total vision throughout the introduction is preferable, keeping the tip always identifiable. Small movements of the needle inclination and consensual adjustments of the probe almost always allow for a good result of the manoeuvre. The target is also previously studied in terms of its dimensions, contour, echogenicity and vascularity, and the access strategy is planned. It is good practice to precede the manoeuvre with good anaesthesia and an increase in Time Gain Compensation (TGC) on the superficial sections to better guide the direction of the needle immediately. The instruments are the same as for normal biopsies,

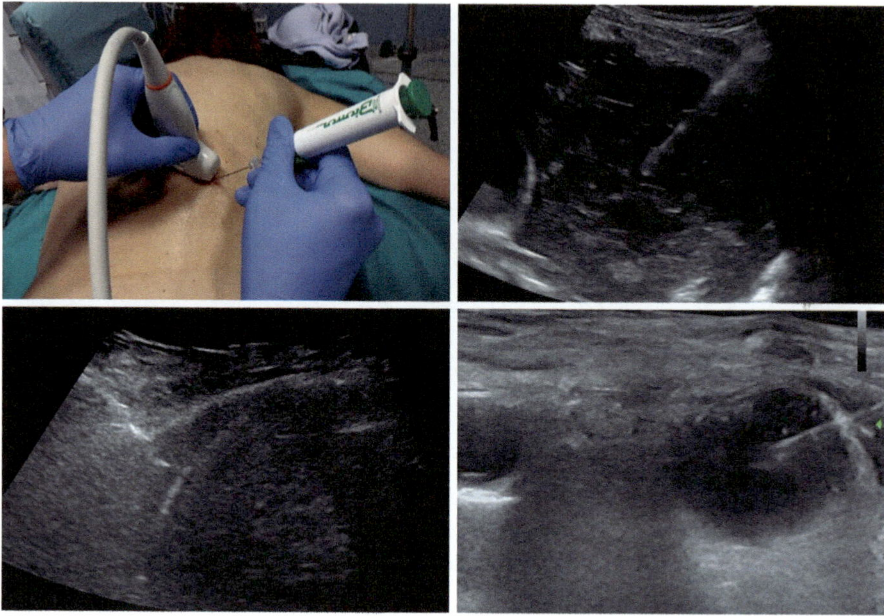

Fig. 18.11 Ultrasound-guided biopsy

small light tru-cuts and manoeuvrable with one hand (the probe in the other), of 21 G if centred on the parenchyma, 18 G if on the chest wall and pleura [21].

All anomalies of the chest, if visible with ultrasound, can be punctured, aiding the diagnosis and staging of pleural diseases. Wall swelling, costal osteolysis, parasternal neoformations and axillary or laterocervical lymph nodes are easily reachable, with very high diagnostic rates.

Finally, ultrasound allows for the identification of any post-procedural complications such as pneumothorax or haemothorax. The diagnostic yield, in expert hands, exceeds 90% [22].

Ultrasound allows for diagnostic thoracoscopy without pleural effusion and with difficult access.

For medical thoracoscopy, the classic methodology involved a preparatory pneumothorax; however, over time ultrasound has gradually replaced this practice, making the examination more incisive and safer (Table 18.2). The presence of fluid in lateral decubitus before the examination is easily detected and the entrance point becomes easy to identify. Ultrasound also provides other preliminary information useful during endoscopy: the involvement of the diaphragm, the presence of masses and/or adhesions that must be avoided during the insertion of the trocar, the state of the lung parenchyma, the Echogeniciy of effusions of the material present and the distribution of the effusion within the thorax (Table 18.2).

Table 18.2 Advantages of echo-guided in medical thoracoscopy

Echo-guided thoracoscopy: advantages
• Pre-endoscopic panorama
• No preparatory pneumothorax
• Measures the amount of liquid
• Defines the arrangement of the liquid
• Predicts the consistency of the liquid
• Enables unusual inputs
• Identifies pockets
• Aids in decision on pleurodesis
• Identifies incarcerated lung
• Finds the diaphragm position
• Plans the exam strategy
• Useful at the post-examination stage

The examination has recently become feasible even in the absence of pleural fluid when it can be essential to perform biopsies on small nodules or thickenings that cannot be reached from the outside or located in difficult locations such as the retroscapular area. A meticulous analysis of the 'sliding' in all quadrants, first in a sitting position where its expression is maximum and then in lateral decubitus, provides valuable information on the collapsibility of the lung. If sliding is present, it is possible to effect a cautious entry using blunt-tipped scissors and subsequent introduction of the trocar (generally 7 mm in diameter in medical thoracoscopy) without producing damage and with the immediate formation of a pleural chamber suitable for exploration and subsequent biopsies. An alternative is the technique of creating the preparatory pneumothorax with blunt needles such as those used by Boutin, introduced into the cavity, always in the presence of sliding, before the introduction of the trocar.

In infectious effusions (◘ Fig. 18.12), ultrasounds become not only useful but indispensable. The pockets of fibrin, present even in the first hours of the disease, are easily identified and monitored. Evolution can be very fast; hence, timely ultrasound is decisive in the strategy to be adopted. If the settings are many and rapidly evolving, the ultrasound guides the timing of the interventions, when to place the drain in the first

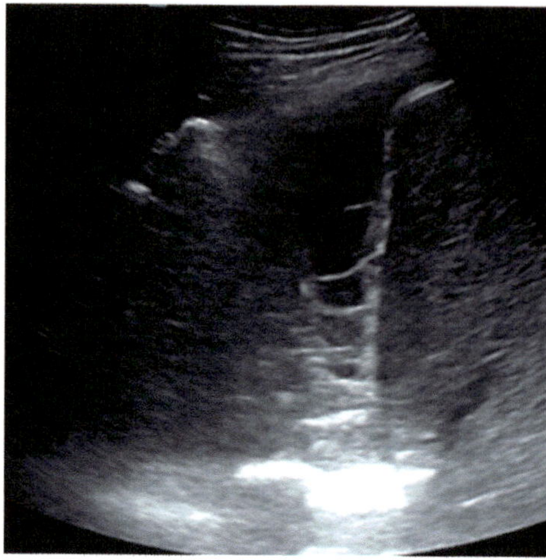
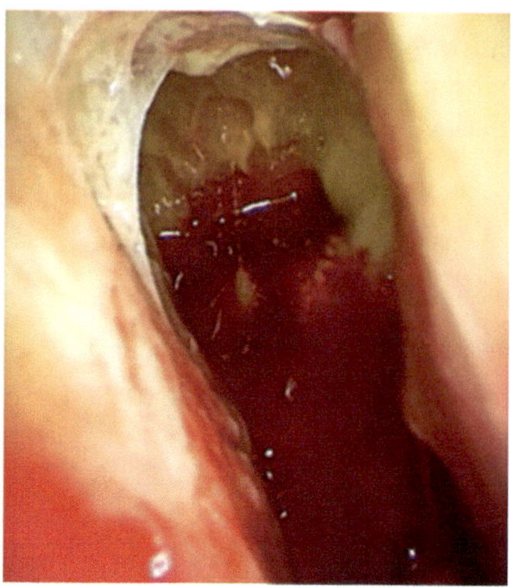

Fig. 18.12 Guided ultrasound thoracoscopy

place but also whether to switch immediately to thoracoscopy with mechanical lavage of the cavity, hence guaranteeing early healing, shorter hospitalisation and reduced recourse to surgery. It also guides the access points in the larger sacs, determining the endoscopic operative strategy.

After the examination, ultrasound enables us to monitor parenchymal re-expansion as well as to control the trend of residual loculations and to guide any fibrinolytic therapy.

Even after pleurodesis, a good ultrasound examination can provide valuable information as to its effectiveness and maintenance over time.

18.7 Conclusions

Ultrasound has made the pulmonologist much more independent of other specialists.

In summary, this chapter is intended as an invitation to the increasingly widespread use of chest ultrasound by the pulmonologist who, if he wishes to rise to the challenge of modernity, must acquire the appropriate skills and technology. Ultrasounds are indicated in any setting, in the ward and in emergencies, in follow-ups and in specialist clinics. The pleura is thus the ideal subject for studying with ultrasound. Historically, it was the first 'organ' widely analysed with ultrasound. The Pulmonologist may have been late in noticing the importance of ultrasound for the examination of the pleura, but is rapidly closing the gap by bringing new and passionate contributions but above all by using it every day in routine clinical activity.

References

1. Joyner CR Jr, Herman RJ, Reid JM. Reflected ultrasound in the detection and localization of pleural effusion. Trans Am Clin Climatol Assoc. 1967;78:28–37. PMID: 6071511.
2. Porcel JM. Pleural ultrasound for clinicians. Rev Clin Esp. 2016;216(8):427–35. https://doi.org/10.1016/j.rce.2016.05.009.
3. Williamson JP, Grainge C, Parameswaran A, Twaddell SH. Thoracic ultrasound: what non-radiologists need to know. Curr Pulm Rep. 2017;6(1):39–47. https://doi.org/10.1007/s13665-017-0164-1.
4. Marchetti G, Valsecchi A, Indellicati D, et al. Ultrasound-guided in medical thoracoscopy in absence of pleural effusion. Chest. 2015;147(4):1008–12. https://doi.org/10.1378/chest.14-0637.
5. Mayo PH, Doelken P. Pleural ultrasonography. Clin Chest Med. 2006;27(2):215–27. https://doi.org/10.1016/j.ccm.2006.01.003.
6. Koenig SJ, Narasimhan M, Mayo PH. Thoracic ultrasonography for the pulmonary specialist. Chest. 2011;140(5):1332–41. https://doi.org/10.1378/chest.11-0348.
7. Lichtenstein DA. The pleural line. Lung ultrasound in the critically ill. Cham: Springer; 2016. https://doi.org/10.1007/978-3-319-15371-1_8.
8. Reuss J. Sonography of the pleura. Ultraschall Med. 2010;31(1):8–22. https://doi.org/10.1055/s-0028-1109995, quiz 23-5. English, German. Epub 2010 Feb 15. PMID: 20157868.
9. Dietrich CF, et al. Ultrasound of the pleurae and lungs. Ultrasound Med Biol. 2015;41(2):351–65. https://doi.org/10.1016/j.ultrasmedbio.2014.10.002.
10. Eibenberger KL, Dock WI, Ammann ME, et al. Quantification of pleural effusions: sonography versus radiography. Radiology. 1994;191(3):681–4. https://doi.org/10.1148/radiology.191.3.8184046.
11. Salamonsen MR, Lo AKC, Ng ACT, Bashirzadeh F, Wang WYS, Fielding DIK. Novel use of pleural ultrasound can identify malignant entrapped lung prior to effusion drainage. Chest. 2014;146(5):1286–93. https://doi.org/10.1378/chest.13-2876. PMID: 25010364.
12. Wernecke K. Ultrasound study of the pleura. Eur Radiol. 2000;10(10):1515–23. https://doi.org/10.1007/s003300000526.
13. Lichtenstein D, Mezière G, Seitz J. The dynamic air bronchogram. A lung ultrasound sign of alveolar consolidation ruling out atelectasis. Chest. 2009;135(6):1421–5. https://doi.org/10.1378/chest.08-2281. Epub 2009 Feb 18. PMID: 19225063.
14. Alrajab S, Youssef AM, Akkus NI, Caldito G. Pleural ultrasonography versus chest radiography for the diagnosis of pneumothorax: review of the literature and meta-analysis. Crit Care. 2013;17(5):R208. https://doi.org/10.1186/cc13016.
15. Lichtenstein DA, Menu Y. A bedside ultrasound sign ruling out pneumothorax in the critically ill. Lung sliding. Chest. 1995;108(5):1345–8. https://doi.org/10.1378/chest.108.5.1345.
16. Morgan RA, Pickworth FE, Dubbins PA, McGavin CR. The ultrasound appearance of asbestos-related pleural plaques. Clin Radiol. 1991;44(6):413–6. https://doi.org/10.1016/s0009-9260(05)80662-2.
17. Saito T, Kobayashi H, Kitamura S. Ultrasonographic approach to diagnosing chest wall tumors. Chest. 1988;94(6):1271–5. https://doi.org/10.1378/chest.94.6.1271.
18. Qureshi NR, Rahman NR, Gleeson FV. Thoracic ultrasound in the diagnosis of malignant pleural effusion. Thorax. 2009;64:139–43. https://doi.org/10.1136/thx.2008.100545.
19. Hooper C, Lee YC, Maskell N, BTS Pleural Guideline Group. Investigation of a unilateral pleural effusion in adults: British Thoracic

Society Pleural Disease Guideline. Thorax. 2010;65(Suppl. 2):ii4–17. https://doi.org/10.1136/thx.2010.136978.

20. Hendin A, Koenig S, Millington SJ. Better with ultrasound: thoracic ultrasound. Chest. 2020;158(5):2082–9. https://doi.org/10.1016/j.chest.2020.04.052. Epub 2020 May 16. PMID: 32422131.
21. Mei F, Bonifazi M, Rota M, Cirilli L, Grilli M, Duranti C, Zuccatosta L, Bedawi EO, McCracken D, Gasparini S, Rahman NM. Diagnostic yield and safety of image-guided pleural biopsy: a systematic review and meta-analysis. Respiration. 2021;100(1):77–87. https://doi.org/10.1159/000511626. Epub 2020 Dec 29. PMID: 33373985.
22. Staub LJ, Biscaro RRM, Kaszubowski E, Maurici R. Chest ultrasonography for the emergency diagnosis of traumatic pneumothorax and haemothorax: a systematic review and meta-analysis. Injury. 2018;49(3):457–66. https://doi.org/10.1016/j.injury.2018.01.033. Epub Feb 8 2018. PMID: 29433802.

Use of Cortisone in Pleural Pathology

Angelo G. Casalini

Contents

A. G. Casalini (ed.), *Practical Manual of Pleural Pathology*,
https://doi.org/10.1007/978-3-031-20312-1_19

A debated topic too often entrusted to choices that do not find confirmation in the scientific literature is that of the use of corticosteroids in the treatment of infectious and non-infectious pleural effusions.

> In infectious pleural effusion, I always add cortisone to the therapy!

> In the effusion which resolves slowly, why don't we add some cortisone to the therapy?

> In my experience, I have always added cortisone and I have seen that it works!

We often hear this type of comment from colleagues dealing with pleural effusions. Unfortunately, in many medical settings, a little cortisone is prescribed to all and sundry! But is there any scientific justification for this behaviour and this therapeutic choice?

Cortisone: yes or no?

Pleural Pathology is very important and does not merit this superficial behaviour! It is not the purpose of this manual to question the experiences of other colleagues; however, very often, these are based on a few anecdotal cases, while our therapeutic choices should always be guided by the most trustworthy scientific literature.

The aim is to follow the authoritative scientific literature.

To address the problem of the use of cortisone in a rational way, it is therefore worth taking a look at the authoritative scientific literature, the most important Guidelines and the Cochrane Library, to find out whether there are real and justified reasons for its use or not; this is the aim of this short chapter.

If we review the causes of pleural effusion reported in Table 1.1 of ► Chap. 1 and analyse them individually, we can exclude the use of cortisone in all transudates; in these effusions, the only therapy is that specific to the disease that causes the effusion. Let us therefore analyse the most frequent exudative effusions, and in particular infectious and tuberculous pleural effusion.

19.1 Infectious Pleural Effusion

We begin by evaluating the most authoritative scientific literature concerning infectious pleural effusion, in particular simple and complicated parapneumonic effusion and empyema. This is certainly the field in which cortisone is most often used in therapy; but is there a clear scientific justification?

If we look for the term 'corticosteroid' (or similar) in the 2010 BTS Pleural Disease Guideline [1], in chapter dedicated to infectious pleural effusion, we find only one citation, which includes cortisone among potentially immunosuppressive drugs, that is, among the possible risk factors for infectious effusions, as is the case for its use in pneumonia [2]. Its use for therapeutic purposes is never indicated!

Corticosteroids are not considered by the BTS GL in infectious pleural effusion.

The use of cortisone in this field probably derives from its use in pneumonia, but also this use is not always shared or justified even in pneumonia. For example, the recent ATS guidelines on Diagnosis and Treatment of Adults with Community-acquired Pneumonia [3] do not recommend its use except in patients with refractory septic shock; even a recent Cochrane review [4] concludes that, although corticosteroids reduce mortality, clinical failure, complication rates, length of hospitalisation and time to clinical cure in adults with severe CAP, they do not reduce mortality in adults and children with non-severe CAP; patients with non-severe CAP may benefit from corticosteroid therapy as well, but with no advantage for survival.

This extension of cortisone therapy from pneumonia to infectious pleural effusions, similarly to what has already been said about antibiotic therapy, is neither correct nor justified. These are two different pathologies with often different aetiologies, and it is therefore essential to keep the two pathologies, infectious pleural effusions and pneumonia, separate and to distinguish the therapy of pneumonia from that of infectious pleural effusions, and not only with regard to the choice of antibiotic therapy! See 'Antibiotic Therapy' in the chapter on infectious pleural effusion.

The only study in the literature to evaluate the efficacy of systemic corticosteroids in parapneumonic effusions was carried out in the paediatric field [5]. It was a multi-centre, double-blind, parallel-group, placebo-controlled clinical trial conducted among 60 randomised patients aged 1 month to 14 years with CAP and pleural effusion (mean age, 4.7 years; 58% female), in which half were treated with dexamethasone (DXM) and the other half with a placebo. Patients were scheduled for eight intravenous doses of DXM, 0.25 mg/kg every 6 h, or the corresponding volume of placebo, over 48 h. Fifty-seven (95%) children completed the study. The result obtained is that in the group treated with DXM there was a shorter duration in recovery time (defined with clinical and radiological criteria), but only in those with simple and uncomplicated pleural effusion. Therefore, the limit of this study is that it does not include complicated pleural effusion and empyema!

There are no clinical studies that demonstrate the usefulness of cortisone in adult patients affected with infectious pleural effusion.

For the adult patient, there are no clinical studies that demonstrate the usefulness of cortisone. In a recent paper [6], the different possible therapies for infectious pleural effusion are considered, but there is no mention of the use of corticosteroids.

A multi-centre clinical study (STOPPE: Steroid Therapy and Outcome of Parapneumonic Pleural Effusions) is underway [7] at the time of going to print; it is the only one in adults to evaluate the real effectiveness of steroid therapy in this field. STOPPE is a multi-centre pilot study, a double-blinded, placebo-controlled RCT that will randomise 80 patients with parapneumonic effusions to intravenous dexamethasone or placebo (2:1), administered twice daily for 48 h. The 2:1 randomisation strategy will include 50+ participants in the dexamethasone arm in order to increase the power of detecting treatment-related adverse events. The endpoints of this study are many: time to clinical stability, inflammatory markers, quality of life, length of hospital stay, proportion of patients requiring escalation of care (thoracostomy or thoracoscopy) and mortality. Safety will be assessed by monitoring for the incidence of adverse events during the study. The protocol states that all patients must have pneumonia with associated pleural effusion. This is a limitation because we must consider that many patients lack evidence of underlying pneumonia [8]; therefore, the so-called 'primitive or primary empyemas', which represent a large number of cases and often have a different aetiology [8], will not be taken into consideration in this study. A recent paper [9] documents that the radiological evidence of pneumonia was present in only 43.8% of 164 community-acquired empyemas. Please refer to the second Clinical Case of Infectious Pleural Effusion in this manual.

If we look in the Cochrane Library for meta-analyses on the use of cortisone drugs in infectious pleurisy, we will be disappointed.

The Cochrane reviews only examine randomised and controlled trials [10] to evaluate the effectiveness of a therapy, and nothing is found in the field of infectious pleural effusion about the use of cortisone.

The 'vocation' of the Cochrane Library to evaluate the effectiveness of cortisone therapy in many fields is well established. The proof is that the Cochrane logo itself (◘ Fig. 19.1) derives from a systematic review of randomised studies, which showed that corticosteroids given prior to pre-term birth (as a result of either pre-term labour or elective pre-term delivery) are effective in preventing respiratory distress syndrome and neonatal mortality [11, 12].

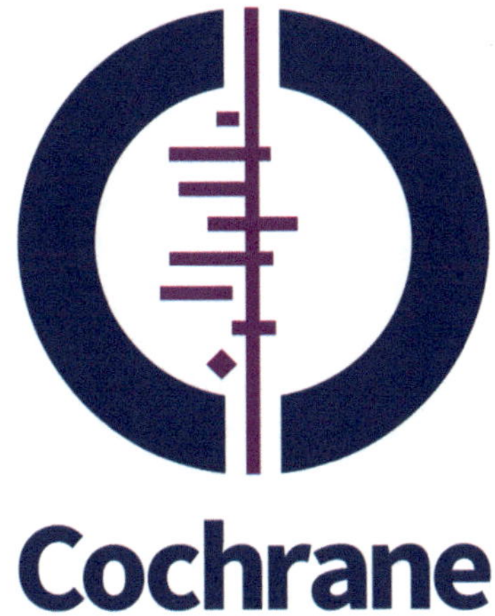

Fig. 19.1 Logo of the Cochrane Library

19.2 Tuberculous Pleural Effusion

Let's see what is found in the literature on the use of cortisone in tuberculous pleural effusion.

In a 2007 Cochrane review on the use of corticosteroids in tuberculous pleurisy [13], the following outcomes were evaluated: death from any cause, improvement in respiratory function, reabsorption of pleural effusion, presence of pleural thickening, presence of pleural adhesions, improvement in clinical symptoms and signs, adverse events and HIV-associated events. The authors' conclusions are that there are insufficient data to recommend their use for the improvement of lung function or to reduce the risk of death. Compared to placebo, adjunctive corticosteroids appear to hasten the reabsorption of pleural fluid, with trials finding an overall reduction of 24% in the risk of residual fluid 4 weeks after the start of treatment. Similarly, there is evidence that corticosteroids reduce the likelihood of pleural thickening at the end of treatment. The authors recommend caution in the use of corticosteroids in HIV patients as the risk of Kaposi's sarcoma was found to be substantially higher in the corticosteroid group; this is a potentially important finding that requires confirmation in future trials. The included randomised controlled trials provide insufficient data to support evidence-based recommendations regarding the use of corticosteroids to reduce the risk of death or for improvement in lung function in participants with tuberculous pleural effusion, regardless of HIV status. There is also no rigorous evidence to support the use of corticosteroids in patients co-infected with HIV, in whom there is some cause for concern that corticosteroids may increase the risk of Kaposi's sarcoma.

The Cochrane review does not provide evidence to recommend the use of corticosteroids in TB pleurisy.

A subsequent Cochrane review in 2017 [14] carefully reviews the same outcomes and cautiously arrives at the same conclusions while pointing out that they have a 'low level of evidence'. This review does not provide enough substantial evidence on patient-important outcomes to recommend the use of corticosteroids in patients with TB pleurisy. The efficacy of corticosteroids in reducing the time to resolution of pleural effusion or symptoms is uncertain, although the included trials that were at low risk of bias did demonstrate more rapid resolution of pleural effusion on chest X-ray in participants treated with corticosteroids. There may be a decreased risk of pleural changes such as pleural thickening and pleural adhesions on chest X-ray at the end of treatment with corticosteroids, but it is unclear how this relates to patient-important outcomes such as disability, lung function and mortality. The concerns raised regarding adverse events in both HIV-negative and HIV-positive patients with pleural TB need to be taken into account when deciding whether or not to use corticosteroids.

The NICE Guidelines published in 2016 [15] do not recommend the use of corticosteroids in tuberculous pleurisy under any circumstances.

Nice Guidelines 2016 and Index TB 2016 do not recommend cortisone in TB pleurisy.

The 2016 Index-TB guidelines [16], like other scientific papers in the literature for the therapy of extrapulmonary tuberculosis [17], recommend the use of cortisones in the therapy of tuberculous meningitis and of tuberculous pericarditis, but do not recommend their use in tuberculous pleurisy.

Light, in the latest version of the Textbook of Pleural Diseases [18], while premising that corticosteroids could reduce the degree of inflammation of the pleura, cites the Cochrane review of 2000 [19] to conclude that there is insufficient evidence to establish that corticosteroids are useful in tuberculous pleurisy. Light [20] and Porcel [21] suggest that in selected patients who continue to have symptoms (particularly fever) after 2 weeks of chemotherapy, a short course of corticosteroids (80 mg prednisone/day until symptoms disappear) may be helpful.

In the literature, there are also curious papers such as a randomised double-blind study from 1988 [22] in which two groups of patients under the age of 45 with tuberculous pleurisy diagnosed with pleural biopsy were compared; steroid therapy was added in the first group, of 21 patients, and placebo in the second, of 19. The study compares the time to reabsorption of pleural fluid between the two groups: 54 days in the group treated with cortisone and 123 in the placebo group; on the basis of this, the authors conclude in favour of steroid therapy. However, it should be emphasised that in all patients only a diagnostic thoracentesis of less than 50 mL was performed, not followed by a therapeutic evacuative thoracentesis! And this is certainly a very questionable diagnostic-therapeutic behaviour! In fact, in two controlled studies in which therapeutical thoracentesis was performed, there were no benefits [23, 24]. According to Sahn, routine use of corticosteroids cannot be recommended and should only be used if acute symptoms, such as fever, chest pain or dyspnoea, are disturbing to the patient [25].

It can therefore be concluded that the decision whether to insert a cortisone therapy or not in a patient with tuberculous pleurisy is left to the expertise and experience of the doctor who will evaluate the possible benefits and any possible side effects, but without forgetting what is present in authoritative scientific literature!

19.3 Other Pleural Effusions

Other pleural effusions for which in some situations there is the indication for the use of cortisone are those in connective tissue diseases. Regarding therapy with cortisone in these pathologies, reference should be made to the specific scientific literature since cortisone therapy could be part of the basic therapy for the pathology in question.

References

1. Davies HE, Davies RJ, Davies CW, BTS Pleural Disease Guideline Group. Management of pleural infection in adults: British Thoracic Society Pleural Disease Guideline 2010. Thorax. 2010;65(Suppl. 2):ii41–53. https://doi.org/10.1136/thx.2010.137000. PMID: 20696693.
2. Maskell NA, Batt S, Hedley EL, Davies CW, Gillespie SH, Davies RJ. The bacteriology of pleural infection by genetic and standard methods and its mortality significance. Am J Respir Crit Care Med. 2006;174(7):817–23. https://doi.org/10.1164/rccm.200601-074OC. Epub 2006 Jul 13. PMID: 16840746.
3. Metlay JP, Waterer GW, Long AC, Anzueto A, Brozek J, Crothers K, Cooley LA, Dean NC, Fine MJ, Flanders SA, Griffin MR, Metersky ML, Musher DM, Restrepo MI, Whitney CG. Diagnosis and Treatment of Adults with Community-acquired Pneumonia. An Official Clinical Practice Guideline of the American Thoracic Society and Infectious Diseases Society of America. Am J Respir Crit Care Med. 2019;200(7):e45–67. https://doi.org/10.1164/rccm.201908-1581ST. PMID: 31573350; PMCID: PMC6812437.
4. Stern A, Skalsky K, Avni T, Carrara E, Leibovici L, Paul M. Corticosteroids for pneumonia. Cochrane Database Syst Rev. 2017;12(12):CD007720. https://doi.org/10.1002/14651858.CD007720.pub3. PMID: 29236286; PMCID: PMC6486210.
5. Tagarro A, Otheo E, Baquero-Artigao F, Navarro ML, Velasco R, Ruiz M, Penín M, Moreno D, Rojo P, Madero R, CORTEEC Study

Group. Dexamethasone for parapneumonic pleural effusion: a randomized, double-blind, clinical trial. J Pediatr. 2017;185:117–123.e6. https://doi.org/10.1016/j.jpeds.2017.02.043. Epub 2017 Mar 28. PMID: 28363363.

6. Sundaralingam A, Banka R, Rahman NM. Management of pleural infection. Pulm Ther. 2021;7(1):59–74. https://doi.org/10.1007/s41030-020-00140-7. Epub 2020 Dec 9. PMID: 33296057; PMCID: PMC7724776.
7. Fitzgerald DB, Waterer GW, Read CA, Fysh ET, Shrestha R, Stanley C, Muruganandan S, Lan NSH, Popowicz ND, Peddle-McIntyre CJ, Rahman NM, Gan SK, Murray K, Lee YCG. Steroid therapy and outcome of parapneumonic pleural effusions (STOPPE): Study protocol for a multicenter, double-blinded, placebo-controlled randomized clinical trial. Medicine (Baltimore). 2019;98(43):e17397. https://doi.org/10.1097/MD.0000000000017397. PMID: 31651842; PMCID: PMC6824804.
8. Dyrhovden R, Nygaard RM, Patel R, Ulvestad E, Kommedal Ø. The bacterial aetiology of pleural empyema. A descriptive and comparative metagenomic study. Clin Microbiol Infect. 2019;25(8):981–6. https://doi.org/10.1016/j.cmi.2018.11.030. Epub 2018 Dec 21. PMID: 30580031.
9. Brims F, Popowicz N, Rosenstengel A, Hart J, Yogendran A, Read CA, Lee F, Shrestha R, Franke A, Lewis JR, Kay I, Waterer G, Lee YCG. Bacteriology and clinical outcomes of patients with culture-positive pleural infection in Western Australia: a 6-year analysis. Respirology. 2019;24(2):171–8. https://doi.org/10.1111/resp.13395. Epub 2018 Sep 6. PMID: 30187976.
10. Stavrou A, Challoumas D, Dimitrakakis G. Archibald Cochrane (1909-1988): the father of evidence-based medicine. Interact Cardiovasc Thorac Surg. 2014;18(1):121–4. https://doi.org/10.1093/icvts/ivt451. Epub 2013 Oct 18. PMID: 24140816; PMCID: PMC3867052.
11. Crowley P, Chalmers I, Keirse MJ. The effects of corticosteroid administration before preterm delivery: an overview of the evidence from controlled trials. Br J Obstet Gynaecol. 1990;97(1):11–25. https://doi.org/10.1111/j.1471-0528.1990.tb01711.x. PMID: 2137711.
12. McGoldrick E, Stewart F, Parker R, Dalziel SR. Antenatal corticosteroids for accelerating fetal lung maturation for women at risk of preterm birth. Cochrane Database Syst Rev. 2020;(12):CD004454. https://doi.org/10.1002/14651858.CD004454.pub4.
13. Engel ME, Matchaba PT, Volmink J. Corticosteroids for tuberculous pleurisy. Cochrane Database Syst Rev. 2007;(4):CD001876. https://doi.org/10.1002/14651858.CD001876.pub2. Update in: Cochrane Database Syst Rev. 2017;3: CD001876. PMID: 17943759.
14. Ryan H, Yoo J, Darsini P. Corticosteroids for tuberculous pleurisy. Cochrane Database Syst Rev. 2017;3(3):CD001876. https://doi.org/10.1002/14651858.CD001876.pub3. PMID: 28290161; PMCID: PMC5461868.
15. Hoppe LE, Kettle R, Eisenhut M, Abubakar I, Guideline Development Group. Tuberculosis--diagnosis, management, prevention, and control: summary of updated NICE guidance. BMJ. 2016;352:h6747. https://doi.org/10.1136/bmj.h6747. PMID: 26762607.
16. Sharma SK, Ryan H, Khaparde S, Sachdeva KS, Singh AD, Mohan A, Sarin R, Paramasivan CN, Kumar P, Nischal N, Khatiwada S, Garner P, Tharyan P. Index-TB guidelines: guidelines on extrapulmonary tuberculosis for India. Indian J Med Res. 2017;145(4):448–63. https://

doi.org/10.4103/ijmr.IJMR_1950_16. PMID: 28862176; PMCID: PMC5663158.
17. Ketata W, Rekik WK, Ayadi H, Kammoun S. Les tuberculoses extrapulmonaires [Extrapulmonary tuberculosis]. Rev Pneumol Clin. 2015;71(2–3):83–92. doi: https://doi.org/10.1016/j.pneumo.2014.04.001. French. Epub 2014 Aug 15. PMID: 25131362.
18. Light RW, Lee YC, editors. Textbook of pleural diseases. 3rd ed. Boca Raton, FL: CRC Press; 2016.
19. Matchaba PT, Volmink J. Steroids for treating tuberculous pleurisy. Cochrane Database Syst Rev. 2000;(2): CD001876. doi: https://doi.org/10.1002/14651858.CD001876. Update in: Cochrane Database Syst Rev. 2007;(4): CD001876. PMID: 10796669.
20. Light RW. Update on tuberculous pleural effusion. Respirology. 2010;15(3):451–8. https://doi.org/10.1111/j.1440-1843.2010.01723.x. Epub 2010 Mar 21. PMID: 20345583.
21. Porcel JM. Tuberculous pleural effusion. Lung. 2009;187(5):263–70. https://doi.org/10.1007/s00408-009-9165-3. Epub 2009 Aug 13. PMID: 19672657.
22. Lee CH, Wang WJ, Lan RS, Tsai YH, Chiang YC. Corticosteroids in the treatment of tuberculous pleurisy. A double-blind, placebo-controlled, randomized study. Chest. 1988;94(6):1256–9. https://doi.org/10.1378/chest.94.6.1256. PMID: 3056661.
23. Galarza I, Cañete C, Granados A, Estopà R, Manresa F. Randomised trial of corticosteroids in the treatment of tuberculous pleurisy. Thorax. 1995;50(12):1305–7. https://doi.org/10.1136/thx.50.12.1305. PMID: 8553306; PMCID: PMC1021356.
24. Wyser C, Walzl G, Smedema JP, Swart F, van Schalkwyk EM, van de Wal BW. Corticosteroids in the treatment of tuberculous pleurisy. A double-blind, placebo-controlled, randomized study. Chest. 1996;110(2):333–8. https://doi.org/10.1378/chest.110.2.333. PMID: 8697829.
25. Cohen M, Sahn SA. Resolution of pleural effusions. Chest. 2001;119(5):1547–62. https://doi.org/10.1378/chest.119.5.1547. PMID: 11348966.

GPSR Compliance

The European Union's (EU) General Product Safety Regulation (GPSR) is a set of rules that requires consumer products to be safe and our obligations to ensure this.

If you have any concerns about our products, you can contact us on ProductSafety@springernature.com

In case Publisher is established outside the EU, the EU authorized representative is:

Springer Nature Customer Service Center GmbH
Europaplatz 3
69115 Heidelberg, Germany

Batch number: 10371042

Printed by Printforce, the Netherlands